CW01472167

The Power of Music

The Power of Music

How Music Connects Us All

SHEKU KANNEH-MASON

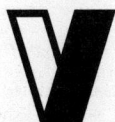

**PENGUIN
VIKING**

VIKING

UK | USA | Canada | Ireland | Australia
India | New Zealand | South Africa

Viking is part of the Penguin Random House group of companies
whose addresses can be found at global.penguinrandomhouse.com.

Penguin Random House UK,
One Embassy Gardens, 8 Viaduct Gardens, London SW11 7BW

penguin.co.uk

Penguin
Random House
UK

First published 2025

001

Set in 13.5/16pt Garamond MT Std
Typeset by Jouve (UK), Milton Keynes
Printed and bound in Great Britain by Clays Ltd, Elcograf S.p.A.

The authorized representative in the EEA is Penguin Random House Ireland,
Morrison Chambers, 32 Nassau Street, Dublin D02 YH68

A CIP catalogue record for this book is available from the British Library

ISBN: 978-0-241-56132-4

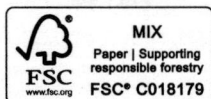

This book is dedicated to my beloved grandfather Arnold Mason
(25 May 1926 – 10 September 2021),
who used to stand in the doorway while I practised,
and who sat and listened to me for hours.

Contents

Foreword

I am a cellist. My reason for writing this book is to examine what that means, and especially what that means for someone like me. When I look at where I'm standing, I realize there were many accidents and surprises paving the way to this position. And also many things in place that steered me in this direction and unsurprisingly, maybe inevitably, led me here.

I want to explore why my first two sentences need the qualifier of 'for someone like me'. My life, at the age of twenty-five, involves regular international concert touring, recording, interviews, television documentaries, work with children and young people, still playing to my conservatoire teacher, Hannah Roberts, and teaching as a professor at the Royal Academy of Music. My live concerts include being a concerto soloist with orchestras across the world, playing chamber music with other musicians I admire, performing recitals with my siblings, practising several hours a day, and constantly working on new repertoire.

I now live in London, but grew up in a noisy house in Nottingham, bulging at the seams with seven children, two parents, lots of instruments, books of music, books in general, board games, art materials, and racks of shoes – mostly football boots and trainers – against the wall by the front and back doors. I went to the local primary and secondary schools in the city, and came home to the smell of big pots of chicken and rice, and the rowdy company of six siblings ready to eat, talk, joke, play and practise. I grew up with music, sharing, play, company and the creative world of imaginative games.

Music existed in a range of contexts and had many manifestations. We danced to music, we sang in choirs, we made up songs together, we listened to music in the car on our way to lessons, or on our way to compete at festivals. We played chamber music together in the hallway, or improvised, bouncing off each other's ideas and knowledge, or simply imitating music we heard on CDs, or the radio, or with our friends. We were taken to classical music concerts at the local concert hall, and listened to other young musicians playing at school, or at Saturday lessons at the Primary and Junior departments of the Royal Academy of Music. We listened to music in church, or on film scores at the cinema, or to accompany stories on CD or tape. And we learnt the art and skill of playing musical instruments.

My parents, although not musicians by profession, had both been taught to play instruments as children. They had seen first-hand how rewarding it was to develop as musicians, and to play with others in orchestras, schools and community groups. They were determined that we should have the same experience.

It was obvious, from an early age, that I would become a cellist. But it was also unlikely that someone like me would become a cellist. It was obvious because, from the moment I had the luck and privilege to hold a cello in my hands, from the moment I was encouraged to learn, it became an overriding preoccupation and the central focus of my days. It was unlikely because I didn't fit the usual profile of a classical cellist. I came from the wrong background. The way I looked and spoke did not fit. I had no evident role model to follow. And that is why a main element of my career as a musician today is the work I do to promote music education. I am passionate about bringing other children and young people from 'likely' or 'unlikely' backgrounds to music, and to introduce them to – or encourage them with – learning to play musical instruments. And this is because I recognize that, even with my family's love of music, it is becoming increasingly unlikely for those with my background to become classical musicians.

The dominant image of a classical musician when I grew up did not look like me. It was difficult to find a projection of who I might be if I became a professional cellist, but the people around me simply refused to admit this was a barrier. I realize now, as an adult, just how effective this refusal was. My parents, relatives and teachers shone their light on the music and not on the world before me. Every child needs the support and encouragement of a family, a community, a school to provide a positive reflection of who they are or might be. Good teaching is vital, and the offer of excellent as well as progressive and in-depth instruction has to be available to all.

I was incredibly lucky to be surrounded by a musical family, musical state schools, a supportive community with many music-making opportunities, and wonderful teachers. But the randomness of luck cannot and should not determine the face and the future of music. Luck is too often the product of unequal privileges, rather than talent, inclination, application or desire. And when luck strikes outside the restrictions of privilege, it's an exception that proves a brutal rule.

I hope I can be an inspiration to those who believe in the importance of music, and to those who dream of the chance to perform, to learn and to create music. I hope I can persuade parents, teachers and policy-makers of the value of music for young people. I hope I can continue to bring live and recorded music to people of all ages.

The future of music, in all its glorious forms, depends on what we offer to children from the earliest age, and on how wide we open our doors in welcome. Music is our self-expression, our identities, our histories, our individual memories and our collective selves. Music is what makes us alive, mindful and connected to each other. Music is what makes us empathetic and insightful. Music is what makes us human. This is the power of music.

1. Influence and Inspiration

One of my earliest, most vivid, memories takes place in the house of my Welsh maternal grandmother, Megan Kanneh. I must have been about five years old and the sun was streaming through the glass doors at the back of the dining room, which we called the 'playroom'. There was an LP turning on the record player, and it was a Bob Marley album. I don't recall which one, but I remember the way his voice made me stand, stock-still, as though time had been arrested and a beautiful space opened up where nothing existed except the music. I was usually running, climbing, wrestling with my brother or racing with my sisters, but now all else dissolved except for this special sound that spoke personally to me. The music had a depth I didn't question, but which I was able to sink into, alert to the way it made me feel, light and heavy at the same time.

Another early memory is in Antigua, in the Caribbean, where we were staying with our Antiguan grandparents, Enid and Arnold Mason, my dad's parents. It was Carnival, early on J'ouvert Morning, and we were standing on the side of the road, grown-ups towering above my six-year-old self, and an incredible energy driving through my body from the rhythm of the steel pans. The first lorry came past and I could finally see what I'd been hearing. The lorry shook and bounced with the dancing, drumming, violent beating of the pans and the song they sang was hammered out through my body with a kind of sweet pain that transfixed me.

Later, at the age of seven, I remember sitting in the family car, crammed full of brother and sisters. It was half-term and my mum was driving us to swimming lessons. Time in the family nine-seater car was always music time, whether we were on the way to piano lessons, or to a music festival competition, or to visit grandparents. We had been listening to Schubert's Piano Quintet in A Major, D.667, known as the 'Trout' Quintet, on repeat for a whole week. We heard the chatter of five voices in the piano, violin, viola, cello and double bass, mimicking each other, joking, teasing, each trying to have the last comment, laughing, debating, talking seriously, questioning, having fun. It made me understand that chamber music is like family life. In the love and safety of those you know intimately, ideas are thrown around, caught, developed and changed in a glorious conversation of lively, individual voices. We loved this piece, and sang out each part. By the time we played it together, years later, we knew the piece intimately, and we were enduringly in love with chamber music.

The 'Trout' Quintet has five movements and is just under three quarters of an hour of classical string chamber music. Chamber music – music for two or more instruments – is written to be played in a room, a chamber, rather than on the stage of a grand concert hall. It is music for a home – albeit usually a great home – where the audience is selective and the atmosphere intimate.

This piece was a favourite of my dad's parents, especially the televised version, filmed by Christopher Nupen in 1969 with Daniel Barenboim (piano), Itzhak Perlman (violin), Pinchas Zukerman (viola), Jacqueline du Pré (cello) and Zubin Mehta (double bass). When my grandparents came to visit us in Nottingham, we would play this, recorded from the television, and Grandad would invariably conduct from the settee. The film followed these five famous musicians as they sourced their instruments, rehearsed, played each other's instruments for fun, grandstanded and exchanged interpretations. The serious tension of a performance about to begin on the stage of Queen Elizabeth Hall infused the performative play backstage with an energy we never forgot. And all this became personal in the presence of Grandad, waving his arms, singing along and smiling.

These different musical influences – reggae, soca and classical – are not ranked in my mind as high and low, or serious and frivolous, but they exist together as part of my musical memory, along with so many others. They unlocked what I mean when I think about the purpose of music. They gave me the keys to experience music viscerally, physically and intellectually, and to associate music with the most vital elements of family, history and love.

Music is an art and a skill, but it also has the power to affect emotion, to express inner feelings and to encourage human connection. From childhood to old age, that sense of creative energy and empathy – the understanding of pain, passion, joy and wonder – are vital elements of healthy emotional maturity. Being introduced to music from the earliest age is a gift. It should, however, not be a privilege, by which I mean a special advantage given as a birthright to a circumscribed group of 'special' recipients. Words like these are slippery and can slide into places we don't mean them to be. Music is special and we should of course treat it as a privilege, but also as a fundamental right not fenced off for only the 'privileged'. Music is at the core of our ability to understand others and to unlock our own articulation of self even before we can express ourselves through the spoken word. Yet, sadly, we are moving ever further into a society where music is torn out of state school education and out of reach of the majority of the population. Learning music as a subject, playing a musical instrument, performing as a professional or teaching music to others is becoming the province of a privileged few.

So what do I mean by music? I am often asked, both in media interviews and in more casual conversations, whether I rank classical music in a higher sphere to all other genres, and why I insist on the relevance of classical music in modern life. For me, it is not the genre that is at stake but what the music demands of the listener or the player.

Music has many functions and contexts, and operates at multiple levels. The meaning within the same piece of music can change repeatedly throughout a person's life. Deeper layers of understanding can emerge with greater levels of competence and knowledge. The power and effects of the same piece of music vary according to context, performer, audience, political or social environment. And, while music can create extraordinary group cohesion, everyone stands in their own place while listening.

If I think about Schubert's 'Trout' Quintet, a piece of music that has followed me from childhood to adulthood, from young learner to professional cellist, it hasn't remained frozen in time, but has changed and matured along with me. My first encounters with the piece were based on an idea of musical interpretation as a kind of light-hearted competition between players. The quintet, in the hands of musicians I admired on-screen, and in the joyous appreciation of my grandparents, was ultimately an extension of family life. As children, we sang the parts we'd memorized, switching between instruments in a fantasy rendition of the real thing, projecting our voices into a future shaped by our determination to perform the music with each other and in public.

We had to grapple with the practical realities of translating what was in our heads through instruments we were trying to learn.

Then there was the problem that our violist, Isata, was also our pianist. I was about nine at the time, which meant that four of us were already playing as a budding string quartet. Isata would have been eleven or twelve, Braimah and Konya on violins would have been around ten and eight, and Jeneba six. Aminata would have been only three years old and Mariatu a baby, or perhaps not yet born. My parents had decided that our ambition for Jeneba to play the double bass wasn't remotely practical. We only saw the perfect idea of five of us playing our dream piece. Our parents could foresee the recurring nightmare of trying to get a huge double bass into an already overcrowded car. They knew that seven children, four or five violins and, at that time, one cello left no room for the coveted double bass. So one cello became two and we were one viola and one double bass short of the Trout 'Quintet'.

Playing with family members is an undeniable joy for us. The ease with which we move between banter, bickering and bouncing off each other makes the process of rehearsal riotous, intense and easy all at the same time. But to play Schubert's 'Trout' Quintet we had to work with viola and double bass players outside our family circle. We now couldn't rely on gestures, visual or verbal shortcuts, shared memories or well-worn jokes. There were different skills to learn. This called for a more formal and responsible engagement with the music and we had to be sharper and more alert to what we had happily taken for granted. In that way, the music expanded its borders and took us to places we hadn't imagined.

I remember moving from my understanding of the 'Trout' Quintet as song and lively chatter to something much deeper and more emotional. The more I explored, the more complexity I found. Somehow, my responsibility to the piece became more than simply child's play. It shifted to the art of communicating playfulness while understanding the sophistication of Schubert's composition. I was no longer a young boy, delighted by music, but a musician occupied with the technicalities of an art form. And my job was to reveal a child's delight.

Our first public performance of Schubert's quintet came when we collaborated with Stephen Upshaw and Chi-chi Nwanoku for a Chineke! Foundation event in 2015. Chineke! Orchestra was inaugurated in that year by Chi-chi Nwanoku as a majority Black and ethnically diverse orchestra, with its first concert at Queen Elizabeth Hall two months after this introductory chamber recital. For the first time, we were delving into the music with professional detail and a level of exposure that charged everything with excitement and a shining level of fear. I was sixteen, Braimah seventeen and Isata nineteen. We were so young: there is a video clip of us that day, and when I watch it back now, I can't help noticing that my voice barely sounds broken. Here we were, our dream about to come true in front of a public audience, with the piece we had part-dreamt since those half-term car trips to swimming lessons.

Was this the same piece of music we sang together as small children? We were about to perform this major classical Romantic piece with these two other Black musicians as part of a statement of intent. We wanted to be visible in the world of core classical music as Black musicians and we hadn't forgotten the famous musicians in the Christopher Nupen film. We hadn't forgotten what tradition we were stepping into and disrupting.

Schubert's 'Trout' Quintet is still at the centre of our chamber repertoire, revisited at different moments in our separate and overlapping solo careers. We have just recorded the piece for our most recent family album with Decca Classics with Edgar Francis and Toby Hughes and it always occupies a special, thrilling place in our hearts. On this album, we return to what the music means for our identities as family members in a line of history and heritage from our grandparents to the present.

As human beings, and as emotionally articulate, social people, we all have the need to be introduced to music from the start of our lives. We need music that operates at the deepest levels of our imagination and stimulates our creative intelligence beyond what is deemed to be appropriate for our age and ability. The underestimation of children is the greatest loss to any society.

We need music to demand thought, encourage learning and application, stir concentration and excite the most profound reaction. We also need music for release, for ritual, for dancing, for fun. We need music for the expression both of individual identity and of ourselves in history. Music should be shared, taught, listened to, played and sung. It should also be explained, discussed, reinvented and played with. It is not a question of 'demystifying' music. But we should not be afraid of giving children the tools to think as well as, and in order to, feel. Music is not passive. Knowledge and education should not be divisive words.

In children's learning, music can be part of an education that stimulates responsive engagement. Music challenges children and adults at the deepest levels of their thoughts and feelings. We are, and need to be, active learners and curious, searching, questioning beings. Music can be a fundamental pathway for this.

Children are incredible.

I still think often about the children I knew at primary school. As a state school with a strong musical ethos, Walter Halls Primary School in Nottingham lit the spark for so many of its city children. Words like 'underprivileged' or 'disadvantaged' would have made no sense to any of us, and we certainly didn't *feel* disadvantaged. We were all ordinary children together. Although there is no such thing as ordinary. I used to love putting on school shows, always at Christmas and often in the summer term as well. A transformation would take place where the children around me brimmed over with talents I didn't know they had. From kicking a football around the playground or making too much noise in the classroom, one of my friends would suddenly sing with a voice so clear and in tune it would astonish me. Or they would act out a character onstage and add their own comic twist. Or I would look on in awe as they dominated the stage with brilliant dance moves.

We would see in each other our possible future selves and they seemed limitless. But then, the state secondary education offered to so many of my fellow primary classmates refused to recognize the shining gifts we had all shared as younger pupils. This led, in so many cases, to a great loss of confidence and a personal and collective deprivation I find difficult to accept.

In state education, children are often permitted – or tolerated – to pursue artistic pursuits, but this is regularly followed by an irritated intolerance of serious creativity in teenagers. In English schools, for example, students are encouraged to study the English Baccalaureate, described as 'a set of subjects at GCSE that keeps young people's options open for further study and future careers'. The list includes English language and literature, maths, the sciences, geography or history, a language – but not music.

If we underestimate the importance of creativity we forget to take childhood seriously. By treating music as frivolous, we condescend to children and limit the possibilities of the adults they could become.

Our family built a determined wall against the chipping away of creative confidence. Music was playtime and fun, but it was also serious. We were expected to work. We knew that instrument-learning demanded daily repetition and practice, even when we didn't feel like it. The rewards were reaped through striving and discipline, and these were attributes that linked us to the world of adults and would help us take our place in that world.

If we had not been attentively listened to and taken seriously, our sense of ourselves as serious musicians, or more generally as people with something to say, would have lapsed and been left behind in childhood sparks that lived for brief moments, then died.

My parents say that you always know when a concept is in crisis when you are called upon to analyse it. And then, in its defence, you have to strip it, pull it apart and try to understand intellectually what you already know instinctively. My parents accepted, without question, that music is a natural and necessary part of the human condition and inherent in human well-being. Yet they also understood its status as an art form, a skill and a study.

Music was natural in my parents' lives because it connected them profoundly to their identity. Childhood, familial, cultural and racial identity were all expressed through music and wordlessly connected their lives to ours. We caught glimpses of emotional connections between our mum and dad when they would dance to music from the 1980s or 1990s, or from their wedding – moments they had shared or lived in parallel. They were from the same generation, met at university at the ages of eighteen and twenty, and had inherited the same, much longer and deeper roots and experiences. My parents loved dancing, and they wanted us to dance. All of this was expressed, in something beyond words, in the music they played in the Nottingham house in which we grew up.

As a young child, my influences were multiple and diverse. They were also indiscriminate. Within my family context, alongside reggae, soca and classical, I heard rap music, Welsh folk music, West African music, country and western, dance-hall, male-voice choirs, R&B, soul and more. I was encouraged to dance, to sing in choirs and to sing in church. It was also seen as natural that all seven of us, brothers and sisters, should play instruments.

The move between listening to music and playing music wasn't ever presented as a question: it came entirely naturally. Music was taken seriously in our home because of its power to create group identities and to recollect emotional bonds. Responding to it by dancing and singing also meant learning how to interpret and produce it. My parents applied the same logic to music as we all do to reading: it would make no sense to learn how to read a book if you didn't also learn how to write.

For my parents, their knowledge of classical music had always also been practical. They grew up in families that couldn't afford trips to concert halls and there was no internet to watch things for free. My mother felt her way through music exams on piano and clarinet, was introduced to some music through her school orchestra, and ran her fingers along scores in one of Newport's music shops. There was music all around her, played by school friends, sung by local choirs, taught by her piano and clarinet teacher. The way in was to play. My dad attended one recital – he was taken by his parents as a young boy – of Daniel Barenboim playing Chopin's Preludes, which was a seismic moment in his life, and listened with his dad to his vinyl collection of great classical artists. Otherwise, it was youth orchestra and cello and piano lessons, and the effect of Barenboim's recital was to make him practise more.

My parents accepted that the paths they were taking wouldn't lead them to careers as musicians. It seemed to them a dream that couldn't withstand the practicality of daylight hours. Classical musicians had different lives and came from different backgrounds, and their goal was only to love music and be able to play the music they loved. The leap between that and becoming musicians was too big, and, particularly for my mother, it required training that simply wasn't available. The reality was that the materials and the instruction on offer would never have been enough. My father's parents could only afford a very cheap cello which, looking at my dad's music reports, was a constant source of irritation to his cello teacher, who couldn't understand why they didn't just buy him a better one. And the two pianos available to my mother at different ages were rescued from being thrown on a rubbish tip, and bought second- or third-hand with money scraped together by her grandparents. Good instruments and high-level tuition are either expensive or won as a result of years of excellent teaching. Ambition is nurtured by exposure, self-identification and a sense of possibility. And they both knew they would have to earn a living within the means and the education they could access. But even so, the music was always important.

Classical music was hugely significant for many reasons. For me and my siblings, the expectation was that we would learn to play instruments to a high technical standard, and we knew that the purpose of this, apart from enjoyment, was to constantly challenge and develop our powers of concentration and our stamina. For our parents, that meant classical technique.

The purpose of technique in instrument-learning is the subject of much confusion in popular culture, films and media. I often hear about young musicians, especially in the classical world, being subjected to a regime of brutal, unforgiving training, where nothing but absolute virtuosity is permitted. People seem to believe that the virtuoso is forged in the fire of unlimited suffering – bleeding fingers, hours of agonizing practice – towards a goal of polished perfection. We were always astonished by this idea.

As we grew up, and as young adults together, we would watch, bemused, the depictions onscreen of what a classical musician is. There are a whole host of films depicting the pursuit of classical music and instrument-learning as a form of torture. There are also numerous cameo descriptions in popular culture and sidelong glances at the classical musician inhabiting a world of unnatural privations and miserable repetition. It's easy for these depictions to slip into horror.

We all swung between fascination and laughter when we watched the film *The Perfection* (2018), which focuses on two cellists in an American music conservatory pursuing the rigorous terror of perfection in their playing. The consequences are gruesomely physical as well as mentally warping. *Whiplash* (2014) is a toe-curlingly brutal film, in which perfecting the art of drumming involves intense bodily pain for the pupil and systematic abuse by the teacher. Even *Shine* (1996), in its loving biographical account of the Australian classical pianist David Helfgott, relies on the dramatic mystification of

Rachmaninov's Third Piano Concerto as a piece of such emotional, physical and intellectual magnitude that it can actually accelerate a mental breakdown.

This experience wasn't something my siblings and I recognized at all, but we were well aware of it from the reactions we got from friends and strangers when we admitted that we played classical music. It was often a reaction that fused pity with horror. But we were encouraged by our parents and teachers to see that the pursuit of advanced technique has to be in the service of the music. What were we trying to achieve if it wasn't the unfettered passage of meaning and emotion, with the musician as interpreter and performer? It wasn't about cruelty or the pursuit of some kind of meaningless perfection, but it was about facility: we had to be able to play, and play well. Our aim was, and still is, always to enable our bodies and minds to find and transmit the voice we have inside. We learnt to engage with what we want to say. And finding that ease in communication involves a training, mental and physical, that begins in childhood.

Classical music is demanding in many ways. It demands the attention of the listener to the multiple subtleties, layers and passions in the piece, and a kind of presence in the moment. It is the performer who makes this possible: they must be able, physically as well as mentally, to find and express what the music demands.

As children, my siblings and I began with short sessions

of learning which grew longer as we did. The first instrument I was introduced to was the piano. I was five when my mother gave me my first proper lesson. I clambered on to the piano stool, a cushion on top to bring my elbows almost to the level of the keyboard. I had already watched my elder sister, Isata, almost three years my senior, finding melodies and sequences in these rows of black and white rectangles. It was a matter of finding the code and breaking in. There were patterns and puzzles to bring to the surface, and I wanted to begin. My mother taught me by linking language to music. She insisted that we learn to read letters and words before we learnt to play and read music. Reading music involved the incantation of names and letters with notes and allowed us more deeply into music's secret system. Reading text was a way of preparing the mind for the patterns and signs of music.

I had to press my right thumb on Middle C, lining it up with my navel. The sound of Middle C was a fixed thing and the other notes, rising higher, D, E, F, G, had their own place in my head and against my fingers. I pressed as hard as I could to make the notes speak and soon learnt the relationship between physical pressure and sound. Mum would point to the shape of the notes on the written stave and each filled black circle, like the point on a graph, was a sound. Soon, its shape determined a measure of time – whether it had a stem, or the type of stem, or was a blank, open minim or semibreve.

Every day, I climbed on to the piano stool to learn the next stage of the language that unfurled before me, and its possibilities very quickly expanded beyond the strict pinning of shapes and names on a page. It was as though the notes lived inside me in their own reality.

One day, Mum and Dad told me to stand with my back to the piano, so that I couldn't see the keys – as they had done with my sister – and played single notes in random order. This was an easy game. I knew all their names instantly. And I knew if they were the black notes in between that were called sharp or flat depending on the tune. My body understood, like a bell vibrating, exactly what the note was and how it felt. Scales and keys held thoughts. They were an inchoate doorway into a mood or a shade of light, or an idea. And music was as natural as breathing.

It was a long time before I understood that this was a rare ability. I simply assumed that everyone had this innate connection to music and everyone could feel and recognize every note instinctually, like orientating yourself in a familiar landscape. Perfect pitch was less common than left-handedness and inherited randomly, and yet it didn't feel random to me.

I had to learn that, however lucky I was to have it, perfect pitch wasn't enough to be a musician. I needed to learn how to tell a story, to describe a mood or a range of ideas through a piece of music and later through an entire recital or concert. This was as rigorous a training as running a marathon and I had to build this ability over time. My muscles – not just in my fingers and arms but in my whole body – had to be strengthened and toned in the right ways to hold an instrument. I had to learn to distribute tension and to finesse the power I needed for each note. I began to see how a series of notes was like a sentence or a phrase, and how poetry and stories were like music. Perhaps that was partly because my mother's passion was for literature and words. She had been a lecturer in English before I was born, and understood music through the language of poetry and narrative. Rhythm and phrasing, for her, made sense through the logic of sentence and utterance, and she was always keen on the phrase, 'But what are you trying to say?'

Learning to play music meant that I had to learn the routine of practice and to understand that I needed to make it happen every day. Improving on an instrument is a balancing act between climbing and not slipping backwards. It is a step-by-step activity that punishes grand leaps to higher crags if you haven't paid attention to the detail along the way. The minutiae of scales and studies helped to train my brain and mind as painstakingly as each turn of fingers and shoulders was training my body. Because I was learning more than one instrument, I had to confront the fundamentals of instinct and machine. I wanted to express what seemed natural inside me through the external tool of the instrument. This is a constant reminder of the relationship between musical knowledge and its mechanical expression. I found moving between piano and cello, for example, and trumpet, trombone, acoustic and bass guitar, as well as between different contexts of playing and learning, a way to challenge complacency. I had to constantly think about the relationship between sound and its production, and I learnt the risks of going into autopilot.

Part of our family routine when we were young was the Sunday afternoon family concert, when we each had to perform a piece, often a work-in-progress, to our siblings and parents. We took this very seriously as there was nowhere to hide and the feedback – given by each person individually – though encouraging and generous, was also searingly honest.

I clearly remember, from the age of seven onwards, walking on to the 'stage' of our narrow hallway at home, in front of the staircase where the 'audience' sat expectantly. Isata would be ready to accompany me on the piano, an upright pushed up against the wall. It was invariably a moment when my heart would beat twice as quickly as usual with excitement and adrenaline, and I was alert with concentration. Ranging up the stairs would be my whole family, even the smallest sisters (I was eleven when my youngest sister, Mariatu, was born, with three siblings in between her and me, and two older than me). Mum and Dad would also sit there, settled in with my brother and sisters, all ready to comment on my playing.

The hushed silence and group scrutiny changed the everyday objects around me – from careworn books and shabby wallpaper, the odd toy and building block in the corner – into the solemn witnesses of an important trial, with me up in the witness box. And yet, I was thrilled by the spotlight, and buzzing with the feeling of everyone's eyes on me. Now was my turn to shine. Now was my turn to reveal what those evenings of scales and scattered passages of music which escaped from the room (often the bathroom) that I practised in, could become. It was the drama of it that I loved, and somehow that drama was at its most intense in that intimate hallway and stairwell, right up close with the people I knew the best.

My love of drama was very useful for bringing life and panache to the music I played – ranging from short transcriptions of great composers when I was six, to movements of sonatas or concertos from the age of nine.

A sonata is a substantial piece, usually in three or four movements, and usually played as a duet with piano. A concerto is a solo piece with orchestra, but can be performed with a piano transcription, in which the piano plays a simplified version of the orchestra score. At this age, I was less willing to focus on the more minute details of the music, instead wanting to showcase my interpretation – the emotion, the bravado, the power of the piece as a whole. Playing without the music was easy and it could let me forget the importance of other details.

A 'fault line' was when I might momentarily lose my place and have a lapse of memory, or make a small mistake – miss an accidental (a sharp or flat, raising or lowering a note by one semitone, a small gap), fumble my notes or go in the wrong direction.

If a fault line occurred in practice or home performance, the rule was that it would definitely appear in any performance elsewhere, or in a competition or exam. A fault line was a warning. If you didn't focus on practising and fixing that mistake, it would lie in wait for you, a wrinkle in the rug to trip you up when you were looking the other way. Of course, I only decided to believe that when it actually happened – which, of course, on several occasions, it did.

Respecting the fault line was part of the balance between confidence and arrogance. You need to develop a brute confidence to perform anything onstage. It's a kind of brash, blind swagger that holds you through the brutality of inspection and appraisal in that searching, public moment. But it has to be tempered with a wash of wakefulness and a determined sense of reality and perspective. The pitfalls are there if you don't watch out for them.

I remember one performance in that hallway when I was swimming gloriously in the fixed attention I was getting as the spotlight performer. All was easy, and I was the source of light – until I wasn't. I felt as though I had been happily flying a kite in the open air, and the air itself had let me down. The music crashed to an earthly stop against the ground and I had lost the ability to make it fly again. In order to recover, I had to learn respect for the earth as well as the air. I had to concentrate on the intellect as well as the heart. I had loosened my concentration on the detail of the piece, and lost my place. Somehow, enjoying the feeling of playing, I had let go of my grip on the score. Drama, passion, emotion and feeling are the drivers of music but you have to be awake to the solidity of detail.

The rule of the fault line was a kind of mantra in the family, and even though I began learning it as a young child, it took me a long time to accept it. I always wanted to find my own way of doing things, and if there was a way to break the rules, or slide unnoticed between them, I would do my best to do so. Children, especially in a group, put a lot of energy into evading surveillance, and we gained an irresistible satisfaction in avoiding as many strictures as we could.

There are many similarities between sport and music. I had friends in school who would have to be at the Nottingham ice rink before the crack of dawn for daily training sessions, while I was practising scales and using the correct fingers at the piano keyboard. I played football as often as I could, and loved the interaction of strategy with physical movement. Football practice and fitness, mental acuity and ball skills, the strength of mind required for peak performance in front of a crowd of parents and friends – these were all linked, for me, to music, and, conversely, I played sport musically, with the skills and habits I'd learnt as a musician. I joined the primary school team and a local club, for which we had to train in all weathers, often in the dark, cold, ice and rain. There was a pattern to decode on the football pitch and an intense alertness to other players. Body strength and control mattered. Regular training, communication and an instinct for planning ahead mattered. And there was the sheer, grinding, competitive determination to succeed.

Fitting football, school, music practice and lessons into a typical week wasn't a feat I worried about or was even particularly conscious of. When it was football training night, I was ready. As soon as the noisy family tea was over, I rushed to pick up my kit and get to the car. At primary school, my brother, Braimah, and I had simply stayed at school and trained with the Sherwood Football Team, which largely overlapped with the school team. Braimah and I were one school year apart, so most of our football and sporting life was spent together. At secondary school, we were members of the same school football team, but had to train apart outside school because of the year's difference. At this stage, between the ages of eleven and sixteen, football training was always a car ride away in rush-hour traffic across Nottingham. It would be too early for my dad to be home from work, so it was Mum's job to take me and pick me up. I lived completely in the present and simply remember running out of the car, ready to play and train, and feeling the same way about matches. I didn't hold back to protect my fingers and arms, I didn't think about practice and homework, and it never occurred to me what other things were being ordered or managed to allow me to play. The routine presented itself as a kind of enabling safety net and I concentrated only on the activity before me, never feeling guilty, or responsible, or having to feel grateful for the creative freedom that gave me.

I loved, and still love, football. But ice skating didn't allow me the same control. I envied the smooth, easy flow that Braimah achieved on the ice and the natural balance he had, it seemed, without thinking. On the ice, I was in a constant battle to gain an equilibrium between body and mind, as though the rug was being repeatedly whipped out from under my feet. I chose football as my sport, and it also chose me.

Music presents similar choices because, in the end, the most meaningful development on an instrument is to choose it, to love it, and to remain dedicated to that choice. The piano fascinated me, and spoke to me, but it was the cello which gave me my voice and which I felt became part of me, because of its set-up which I could feel so close to my own body. I liked the physical proximity of the cello. I liked the way I could hold it with the belly of the sound against my chest and abdomen. When I breathed, the cello breathed, and when I drew the bow across the front, I seemed to exhale its voice through my own body. Any technical challenges felt directly physical. Lunging through a slide – a portamento – to hit a high note was very much like doing a slide tackle to kick a football, and involved risk and precision in perfect balance. That merging of instrument and body comes, not just through a kind of emotional recognition – which is important – but through the physical repetition of exercises, learning to present short pieces with as much attentiveness as possible before becoming more ambitious. It takes a serious approach to accuracy in tuning, tone and timing.

Most children who begin to learn the cello begin with pizzicato – plucking the strings and leaving the bow to one side. This focuses attention on pitch. Each string has its own, fixed sound, separated by an interval of a fifth. Each note in basic music theory exists within a scale, a range of eight notes, that brings you back to the first, an octave (eight notes) higher. Every scale lives in a key, major or minor, with an interval, either a tone or a semitone, between each note. Orchestral stringed instruments, like cello, violin, viola and bass, have strings tuned in fixed intervals, and notes can be raised or lowered by the fingers pressing down in different places, or with differing pressure on each string. With pizzicato, I discovered that the right index finger pulling at each string creates a vibration through the body of the cello, resonating through the F-holes in the front, and down into the floor through the spike at the bottom. As a six-year-old, hugging my quarter-size cello, the thrill was immediate.

Sound reverberated through the wood at the front and at the back, into my chest, into my ribcage and in the sides along my arms. I leant my head close to the fingerboard to hear that rasp of skin against the tough, metal string as I released the tension and freed the sound waves. I soon learnt the relationship between pressure and sound – the gentle, slower movement of the arm for a narrower vibration, and the violent, rounder gesture for a more urgent, louder sound. The use of the left-hand fingers to change the pitch of each string had its own technique. Moving the left arm to the optimum position for weight without tension, learning the correct gaps between each pressed finger for the right tuning, and coordinating right and left hand, were all steps that had to be taken.

And then the bow. Simply registering the weight of the bow in your right hand is a surprise. Its heaviness has to be divided between relaxed thumb and spaced fingers. The liquid movement of wrist, arm and 'soft' shoulder, the application of body weight on particular parts of the bow – tip, middle, heel – and understanding when to apply and release pressure, are all elements of bow technique. Whether to move the arm quickly or slowly – while coordinating the two hands – these are experiments practised through the lifetime of any cellist. As I learnt to handle the mechanics of the cello, I came to understand the links between body and sound, between self and voice, and between exertion and music. And finding these connections begins in childhood.

Playing the cello is not just about physically playing it, but about discovering tonality and keys, the history behind the music, the conventions inherent within it. Every language exists in its own systems of culture, era, tradition and meaning, and music is no exception.

My siblings and I painstakingly learnt the language of Western classical music theory, grew our understanding of how notes on a page translated into live music. We followed scores to see before us, in lines of glorious depth, how music from separate orchestral instruments built into the chorus of an orchestra. The individual voice, honed by practice, joined together with others to create something dynamic and overwhelming in orchestral, chamber and duo performance. This could be broken down into elements, but the finished product – often astounding – could not ultimately be explained. And that was my step into the extraordinary, even the sublime. The outcome – music – was larger than the sum of its parts.

*

I learnt, from a very young age, that music was something I could be part of and never stop learning, but that it would always be more vast and fascinating than I had anticipated. I learnt to be encouraged and motivated, to feel that the music belonged to me, but at the same time to always feel greater and greater astonishment in the face of it. Instead of diminishing, as I grew as a player my sense of awe simply increased.

And, of course, my growth as a player was made possible and carefully nurtured by the skill and care of my cello teachers. I was incredibly lucky to be taught by three different teachers across the years of my learning, from the very beginning and on to postgraduate lessons. Each teacher was able to guide and teach me in the way I needed to be taught, at different ages and stages. I revere the skill of a teacher and recognize the importance of teaching as a profession – it is a vocation honed from years of training, experience and deep understanding of both the instrument and the individual student, whether they're a child, a young person or an adult. My very first cello teacher, Sarah Huson (now Huson-Whyte), had the complex task of teaching me the basic fundamentals of playing the cello, such as how to hold the bow, how to produce the kind of sound that could fill a room, accurate tuning and comfortable posture, while also pushing me forward all the time with new skills, new pieces and more advanced technique. All the while also repeatedly reminding me of the fundamentals; it must have taken enormous diligence.

Professional players have to work hard to reconstruct that feeling of discomfort, and having to concentrate on many new things at once, that all instrument-learners face as students. Trying to explain to a child or new learner how to control all these different things at once in order to make music is not easy. Sarah had to translate the skills she'd harnessed across years of playing and studying – skills which now came naturally to her – to me, an excited child, bewildered by several demands made all at once and all needing attention at the same time. If I focused on the shape of my left hand on the fingerboard, I would forget the bow-hold. If I listened to the tuning, I would forget the speed or position of the bow. My feet, the movement of my arm, the act of reading the notes and keys accurately, listening to the piano part, all these lessons have to be taught, and taught again, and taught in clusters. The key for Sarah was not to let anything, once taught in detail, to pass by or to be effaced by the next thing. Sarah's patience, dynamism and faith in me, while always talking about the music, was an extraordinary start for a six-year-old, and took me all the way to my successful audition for Primary Royal Academy at the age of nine.

My second teacher, Ben Davies, approached teaching as an intensively creative project. How to learn something, whether technique or a musical phrase, was presented through my imagination and he was constantly approaching a piece in different ways. Nothing was ever settled, and I couldn't be lazy about any aspect of my playing. If I hadn't mastered a concept by the next lesson, he immediately jumped on that complacency or lack of practice. There was nowhere I could hide, and I was challenged and pushed into exploring, musically and through experiment, everything I came across.

My next teacher, Hannah Roberts, who I went to as both an undergraduate and a postgraduate at the Royal Academy of Music, is also an extraordinarily imaginative teacher. She has a limitless supply of words she can use to describe what is happening, or should be happening, in the sound I am making and in the feeling that the music demands. Hannah communicates this through images, textures, colours and funny stories. Like Ben, she offers a wealth of analogies to illustrate her ideas, and encourages me to approach music through a deluge of possibilities and senses, keeping my mind and body alive through the cello. The more random, weird or hilarious the analogy is the more you remember it. It is Hannah who has shaped my cello-playing and my musicality, transforming me from an eighteen-year-old boy to the concert cellist and recording artist I now am.

This progression through different teachers and teaching methods remains in the layers that make up my approach to music and the cello, and the learning never ends. I still communicate with, ask advice from, and play to and with all my teachers, and I still have lessons with Hannah. A musician is never a finished artefact, and I am always moving, growing and listening.

I think one of the greatest gifts my parents gave me was to place the rigours and beauty of classical technique and the deep riches of classical music right next to the music of other genres. For us, there was no hierarchy of 'high' and 'low' art, and therefore, who had a right to 'own' classical music was not an issue. As I grew older, I heard these arguments and understood that my own identity was at a fraught cultural and historical nexus of competing political voices. However, as a child, I was given the tools to listen and I was given the permission to play. I use the word 'permission' because outside our home, on the streets, on television, it was clear that playing classical cello and listening to classical music wasn't an obvious choice for someone from my background. Even to have the choice seemed unusual. I felt myself pushing up against a cultural wall while forging my way through the music I played, but the path had already been laid by my elder brother and sister, and opened by my parents and grandparents. I also never felt I had to choose. Classical and non-classical lived side-by-side.

One of the critical, most defining factors in introducing music to children is the music that comes into the home and into the family environment. For us seven children, this happened through the records and CDs our parents loved, played loudly at mealtimes or at times when we danced or sang together. That's when I heard Bob Marley, whose music exists on so many levels and has sustained my listening always. The musical arrangements and the richness of the instrumentation in his songs reveals that interplay of harmony and reaction that is both grass roots and complex. The music changes over time but it's the significance of that individual voice and the meaning it conveys that has been a big influence on me. You can't mistake Bob Marley's voice. It cuts and soars in and over the music – it *is* the music – in a way that can't be imitated. It has a force and an immediacy that is lodged in its own guttural, clear sound. His voice unites, persuades, implores and affects beyond the reach of the words – and through the words. Bob Marley helped me to understand the significance of artistic voice and expression. Music is not communicated as a kind of robotic conduit, but lives in the voice of the artist or soloist.

With Bob Marley, I initially loved the rhythms and harmonies, but then later I understood, more and more, what it was expressing and where it was speaking from. I listened to the sense of enduring struggle and the heaviness of a history of slavery and oppression, as well as expressions of love and community, and felt my place within that. But Bob Marley was not the only musician who made me feel this way. Another huge influence was Elgar's cello concerto, particularly the Jacqueline du Pré recordings. In this concerto, the human expression of grief, anger, darkness and hope also comes with a weight of history that I felt before I even partly understood. And it was Elgar's music through the powerful, individual voice of Jacqueline du Pré's cello that forcefully stirred my imagination.

As a child, I watched Jacqueline du Pré's 1967 performance of the Elgar concerto in the filmed recording with Daniel Barenboim conducting the Philharmonia Orchestra. I heard the music through that first chord on the cello, blasting through the orchestra with a great roar of emotion in the opening phrase. The profound expression – the protest – of grief is there in the written notation. But it lives differently, particularly, additionally, in the performance – physical, intellectual, conscious and unconscious – of Jacqueline du Pré. As with Bob Marley, this was how I understood the importance of the performer as the living voice of the music. Jacqueline du Pré was able to fill her cello sound with a force of personality and feeling that stopped me in my tracks and made me listen – and watch – with all my attention.

I would imitate her playing on my quarter-size, and then my half-size, cello, trying to act out and embody the sound she made. I learnt how to make a vibrato with my left hand and arm by watching her hand oscillate as she pressed the string. It changed the vibration and played with the pitch, as though teasing and drawing the senses to an elusive, meaningful centre that warped and pulled at the emotions. I discovered that slow, fast, wide or narrow vibrato created different sounds and emotions, and moving between them formed the story of a piece. At a similar time in my life, I also discovered that speeding up, slowing down, playing with, and almost dancing with a ball on the football pitch was as important as tearing along at full speed with an explosive kick. All moods and turns mattered within music and came with the balance of time.

As with many of Bob Marley's songs, there are two different recorded versions of Jacqueline du Pré playing Elgar's concerto. There are the different conductors (John Barbirolli and Daniel Barenboim) and orchestras, an audience that's live, digital, audio and/or visual. And the concerto has been recorded multiple times by other artists and is played live by many soloists, orchestras and conductors. Elgar's concerto is not simply one thing, but many. Every performance, whether live or recorded, lives in the interaction of all its collaborators, and in the ears, eyes, minds and hearts of every member of its audience.

By listening to the music, we take on all or some of these elements of meaning, which change over time, or via the individual who is hearing it. We ascribe meaning, we respond with our own emotional capacity and influence. I have played the piece many times and, to date, recorded it once with Simon Rattle and the London Symphony Orchestra. But it is never fixed in me. A great piece, with all its influence from childhood onwards, is a restless, churning, growing thing. And for it to have been given to me when I was so young, and then to have the opportunity to keep learning it, and performing it, is an unspeakable joy.

This is also the case with Bob Marley's music. As a cellist and performer, it is natural for me to play, and it is natural for me to play the music I love. The classical technique I was taught has given me the tools to recreate Bob Marley's music for the cello and to lend my voice to the music through my own arrangements and instinctual understanding. I am able to revisit the music I associate with my earliest memories and to listen again, to recreate it anew. If we give music to children, it lives for ever.

Recordings are extremely important, and bring music to those who could not otherwise hear it. But seeing and hearing music live brings another, immeasurably valuable dimension. I am a passionate proponent of live music in every sense. Learning to be an active listener comes from being in its presence, from active demonstration or live concerts. Music should be a very real, very immediate experience.

In 2020, when the concert halls closed down, when smaller groups of musicians could only perform, shakily and through self-recording, online, when listening and watching an artist or an orchestra play could only happen onscreen, the importance of live performance became agonizingly apparent. I was lucky enough to spend those long lockdowns with seven other musicians, including all of my siblings and Plínio Fernandes, a good friend and talented guitarist who was unable to make it back to his home in Brazil – but I recognize how fortunate this was, and how difficult music-making could have been otherwise. After the pandemic, I realized how much the separation from a wider social and school network had decreased the self-confidence of my youngest sisters. We were all able to play together as a family, and lived at home in a lively crowd while the world shut down around us, but being cut off from musical, as well as social, peers for an extended period of time can have lingering effects. Music is part of social language, and a major part of how we communicate with each other and express ourselves. My second cello teacher, Ben Davies, who taught me from the age of nine to the age of eighteen, says that I didn't actually speak to him at all in the first few years, but spoke volumes through the cello. That's how I learnt to be articulate. That's how I discovered how to say what I really meant.

As children, we were able to see concerts with the biggest names in classical music at the Royal Concert Hall in Nottingham, but only because the events manager, Neil Bennison, launched a scheme for those under the age of twenty-five to watch concerts for only five pounds. There, I learnt about the interpretation of music, and how every performance was a living thing, transformed by artist, audience, conductor, orchestra. I saw the power that each individual musician had, and the overwhelming energy of concentration in the moment that had to be committed to by everyone, including the audience.

Concerts can be incredibly inclusive if children are given access and are welcomed through the door. But children also need the personal welcome. I see it as recognition. By that, I mean that children need to know the music is for them as much as it is for adults and professionals. And that whether playing or listening, any stage of learning, however nascent and new, is celebrated. We, as children of parents who were dedicated to giving us as much access to music as they could afford – and beyond what they could afford – were lucky to have that face-to-face recognition. We were recognized as individuals who could learn to read music, to listen to it, and to play it. There was no doubt, no condescension, and therefore no acceptance of half-measures. *Of course*, the music belonged to us, and we could own it, no less than any child more privileged than us.

Something I remember with great clarity is the visit by the cellist Guy Johnston to Southwell when I was about eight years old. My teacher, Sarah Huson-Whyte, invited him to play Haydn's Cello Concerto in C with her group of young pupils and other young string players, and to give us budding cellists short masterclasses. I had never attended a masterclass before and I was simply fascinated to be in the presence of a cellist who had won BBC

Young Musician and was travelling and performing as a high-profile concert cellist. The excitement we all felt was palpable and I could barely sleep the night before, hardly daring to believe that a real concert cellist was going to be in our midst. That he would listen to us play and even perform with us, was simply amazing. I have never forgotten the experience. The masterclass took place in a room at Southwell Minster, and each of us young cellists walked up in turn to perform to each other and the audience of parents and relatives. I played 'Prayer' by Bloch, an intensely beautiful meditation that allowed me to use the vibrato I had practised and sink deeply into the expression of emotion I was sure the piece needed. I remember the respect with which Guy talked with us all about what we had played, and how. I still retain the advice he gave me and can hear his demonstrations on his own cello. Next to mine, it was gloriously bigger and gloriously richer in sound. It reminded me of the scene in *The Lion King* when Simba tries his childish roar and Mufasa charges in with a grown-up sound that makes the rocks tremble. I was in awe and hoped I could make that sound one day.

During the day, Guy neither conceded to us nor patronized us. Talking to us, he always gave us the space to imagine the music for ourselves. One of the qualities of his teaching was to push and facilitate our own imagination, to encourage and to challenge us. We rehearsed the concerto, with him as soloist and us as his small chamber orchestra, and he simply expected us to play with him.

I remember watching him intently from close proximity as he played. I was focusing fiercely on keeping up and playing in tune. I wanted to be part of his performance and felt myself raising my game to join him, utterly thrilled if he threw a glance my way and urged me on. Anything could happen. It was a lurching, roller-coaster ride, and very exciting, tinged with a keen sense of responsibility and fear. By the time we had got through the adrenaline-fuelled third movement and Guy had finished with us on the triumphant flourish of the last chords, I knew what I wanted my career to be.

Not all of us in that group became professional cellists, but none of us forgot what it was like to be listened to and to be treated as fellow musicians. Because there was no limit to what was expected of me in music, I also learnt to accept no limits in myself.

Nine years later, when I myself won BBC Young Musician at the age of seventeen, Guy Johnston offered to share a concert with me, my sister Jeneba, and the two cello teachers I had learnt from up to this point – Sarah Huson-Whyte and Ben Davies – in what had originally been meant to be his own solo recital at the Playhouse, in my home town of Nottingham. In addition, a coach full of pupils from my school, Trinity, formed part of the celebratory audience. It was active permission for me to share the same stage as a professional cellist who had also won BBC Young Musician in earlier years, and who, in that generosity, wanted to include all that I was and where I had come from. This invitation and this welcome at that time were invaluable to me.

This model of limitless expectation lies behind my parents' approach to children and music and it has two sides. One is to bring music to children on their own terms, while at the same time revealing its endless possibilities. Participation in music can be bilingual or multilingual. We listened to endless nursery rhymes, their songs with simple cadences, harmonies and words, while also being plunged, on the same day, into the vast turbulence of Sibelius's violin concerto. We adored Dame Edna Everage and the Melbourne Symphony Orchestra in their rendition of *Peter and the Wolf* at breakfast time, and listened to Rachmaninov's Second Piano Concerto at teatime. Listening to music is like building with blocks, but they don't have to be placed in order. There's much to be said for throwing the door open to participation in music regardless of its so-called simplicity or difficulty.

Nowadays, music is available online on many platforms. Music is cheap or free in digital spaces. This brings the opportunity of sampling great performances and of hearing music from anywhere in the world by the most, or the least, famous musicians. We should not assume the packaged version is the same thing as the live or the face-to-face. A huge amount of learning can happen online, as well as a significant amount of access to the kind of music that was closed to so many people in the past. But we need to be careful of another form of retrenchment and dispossession. Live spaces are not only for those who feel they belong there because of their background, or cultural acumen or financial means. For classical music in particular, we need to keep democratizing our live performances. This means not only making sure anyone is welcomed into our performance spaces, but also given access – and that can only happen by teaching children the language of this music. That doesn't happen by attempting to strip it of its cultural and historical reference points, but by a greater understanding of what these are, and that they are many and complex.

I was taught to listen to the language of music by being invited to hear it live, and by being expected to engage with the complicated technique of playing it myself. Doors were not shut to certain kinds of music, or to certain kinds of musical language. This doesn't mean that everyone can learn to play everything, but it does mean that we can engage in, appreciate and enjoy music by gaining entry to it, without being burdened by a sense of the forbidden, or of our own, hopeless inadequacy. When we watch a football game, a tennis match or an Olympic sport, whether live or at home on television, most people are not offended by the rare prowess and achievements of the athletes before them. We are encouraged to feel admiration, and to delight in the entertainment that hard work and dedication can display. We are invited to feel inspired in our amateur pursuits, or simply to light a small candle of endeavour in our own lives. In the same way that football is the 'beautiful game', not just for the elite sportspeople in front of us, but for anyone and everyone, elite artists and musicians open a small, bright window on to what is incredible, wonderful and human in all of us.

2. The Power of Chamber Music

As young children, Isata, Braimah and I were invited to appear on the television programme *Yo Gabba Gabba!* which was not a programme about classical music at all, but about anything and everything potentially interesting to other young children. We were placed in the segment named 'Doing Things Together as a Family', which could mean anything at all, and usually did. Although not dedicated to music, or to any activity in particular, this section of the programme did celebrate family relationships and spending time with family, which made complete sense to us. And as our living concept of family life was inextricably tied to music-making, that's what we did.

I was around eight years old, Braimah was nine or ten and Isata was eleven. The television crew came to the Primary Royal Academy of Music where, as a family of musical children, we had been recommended by its inspirational director, Krystyna Budzynska. It was an exciting day out and our first foray into the world of cameras and television studios, our first taste of what it was like to be fussed over, dressed, and expected to get on with it while the cameras swung in our direction. But in fact, we were most excited by the free biscuits and juice in the dressing room. The moment of performance was surreal. We had decided to play Haydn's 'Gypsy Rondo' from Piano Trio No. 39, the lively third movement that demands a strong sense of rhythm and dance, all having to play fast notes and keep a close eye and ear on what the other two were doing.

We have a video of our performance from that day, and my mother says we still play in a very similar way now to how we each played then. I think she's referring to our habits when interacting with each other, reacting to a movement or mannerism from one to the other. Even our musical and facial expressions, she says, were formed already. It's very difficult to extricate our chamber music personalities – created alongside each other in a family where there was lots of time for play of all sorts – from ourselves as adult musicians. I can see the seriousness of our intent as we play. Isata is determined and brilliant, already firm in her acknowledgement of the role of pianist to lay the intricate and virtuosic foundations and glancing at us almost ferociously as she drums out an insistent pace with her fingers. Braimah is clear and melodic, his tuning exact and his violin precise as a song, characteristically furrowing his brow in concentration as his fingers show off their natural ease. I, meanwhile, quirky and instinctive, am darting my eyes from sister to brother, resolved to keep up and shine just as brightly, willing the cello to join in as an equal partner while every twitch and turn of my expression reveals that I'm ready for anything.

Eleven years later, aged nineteen, I walked to the chair that had been put out ready for me between the flowered, ancient arches of St George's Chapel at Windsor Castle. The bride and groom had been escorted to the North Quire Aisle of the Chapel to sign the register and it was my turn to fill the lenses of the television cameras that were beaming the service to a live global audience of more than two billion viewers. This was the royal wedding of Prince Harry and Meghan Markle on 19 May 2018, and my task was to perform three solo pieces with the orchestra, made up of musicians from the BBC National Orchestra of Wales, the English Chamber Orchestra and the Philharmonia.

I have deliberately put these two memories one after the other, not to emphasize a contrast, but to reveal the links. The second memory – being the solo cellist at a royal wedding – is inextricably related to the first memory, of playing with my brother and sister as young children. The experiences and skills I developed in childhood, and the qualities I came to treasure, all carried me to that chair and that moment under the central, decorated arch of St George's Chapel, with the eyes of the world upon me.

There are many images of the stand-out soloist in classical music. From the age of six I watched videos and films of the concert cellist walking out onstage in front of the waiting orchestra, greeted by the conductor in white tie and tailcoat and by a glittering audience holding its collective breath. In this image, the soloist is the main event and prime focal point, and it's all about them. I watched Jacqueline du Pré or Mstislav Rostropovich, for example, sweep or stride to their waiting stool and make their musical statement, lauded by the crowd. The authority and lone call of the soloist dominated the scene for me and I began dreaming myself into that picture.

But here, walking to my chair in front of a congregation of senior royalty, Hollywood stars and celebrities, the atmosphere was hushed and intimate. The small orchestra was arranged to my left and the conductor, Christopher Warren-Green, waited in the charged and thrilling pause as I sat and placed the cello spike into the floor. In this moment, I wasn't relying on drama and pomp, or the glorious role of the individual artist at the dazzling core of the action in the way I had imagined as a child. My job was far simpler and yet far more complex. Everything was scaled down to this personal interconnection of my solo line with a group of players within touching distance, and a conductor watching, managing and corralling everyone together. I needed to listen as much as perform, respond as well as play out the melody and song of the pieces. Each one of my lonely, soaring, expressive phrases or passages had its backup in the orchestra and was consolidated by the conductor. This was call-and-response, and more like the solo singer with the essential community context of the chorus. Music is not selfish and I was not alone.

The reality of the audience was right there in front of me. It would have been impossible to conceptualize more than two billion worldwide viewers and I never tried. This music had a personal message of intense emotion and relied on the quietness of that chapel and the close proximity of the people. I was connecting with and communicating to the people in the present and in my presence.

The vision of the legendary soloist that inspired my cello-playing as a child is a tale of overwhelming attraction, but it can never be the whole story. Practising is, after all, an exercise in aloneness, and it involves the great art of pitting yourself against yourself. Demanding your own unwinking spotlight, practice is solipsistic and self-centred. It is demanding and intense. This ability to carry the burden of musical responsibility is a vital element of a musician's expertise. Your instrumental voice matters. The story which you are burning to tell matters, and it's up to you to tell it faithfully, and with the clarity and beauty of your technique. But the art of telling that story is rarely a solitary one.

Playing a concerto places the soloist as the main player of the theme and the driver of the piece. Often, composers create space for cadenza moments where the soloist can grandstand and play virtuosic and impressive passages without any orchestral accompaniment. The orchestra introduces the soloist with a great cadence of chords for these moments, and will accompany or echo the soloist at other moments. As a concerto soloist, I know I enter the stage with an entire orchestra of instruments behind and around me. I have to interact with the orchestra and the conductor, and really listen to the instruments and rely on everyone listening to me. If I went spiralling off on my own, the whole thing would fall apart.

One important lesson I had to learn as a young cellist was what it really means to perform a sonata. I'm rarely on the stage alone: pieces written for solo cello generally need a piano accompaniment, and cello sonatas are written with piano parts. Because of this, young players often assume a sonata is a solo with a piano accompanist as background assistant to the soloist's strutting glory. They see the pianist as a reflection of themselves, merely echoing or facilitating their prowess without stealing their limelight. I was wrong. In a cello sonata, cello and piano are in equal voice, and the term 'Sonata for cello and piano', or 'Sonata for piano and cello', means just that. The clue is in the 'and'. In fact, in many sonatas, piano pushes for paramount position, which can be disconcerting for a cellist used to taking centre stage. My sonata pianist usually was Isata, and usually still is, and playing concert tours together has long been a big part of our lives. This has always been an invaluable pairing for me. If your pianist is your elder sister, one step ahead of you in age, training, experience and advancement, and ready at all times with an arched eyebrow or witty comment to put you in your place, you can't forget that the sonata isn't a solo effort. We often find ourselves in energetic conversation and teasing battle when we play sonatas together, and, especially with classical sonatas, the piano is garrulous and unstoppable.

I have played concerts and concert tours as a soloist without any accompaniment. I play solo music by J. S. Bach, Benjamin Britten, Gaspar Cassadó, Gwilym Simcock, Leo Brouwer and Edmund Finnis, all composers who have written for unaccompanied cello. I also play my own arrangements of Bob Marley and Aretha Franklin. These concerts demand more than myself as a focal point and I have to feel and hear the different voices in the layered lines of the chords and notes I play. That sense of different voices in harmony or struggle imbues the unaccompanied music I interpret on the cello and it's there in the score. When I play my own versions of Bob Marley or Aretha Franklin, for example, the music in my head and under my bow is a voice and guitar or band, and a history and community of expression. Even in the moments where I as a soloist occupy the stage on my own, the music I play often invokes conversation, chorus or even cacophony in its tones, phrases, chords and repetitions. Part and parcel of my job as a soloist is to hold and express the linear or circular time of stories, contradictions, harmonies and moods in my single body and instrument, not as one person but with the voice of many.

A prime example of this fracturing of the solitary voice is in the music of J. S. Bach's cello suites, which are something of a rite of passage for any budding cellist. Anyone learning to play Bach enters the world of several voices, often coming together in the chordal or sequential harmonies that round the phrases, but also in a kind of emotional, experimental war of restless change, shadow-and-shade, disharmony and tonal disquiet. We, as cellists, not only have to hear and make space for this jostle of voices in our musical understanding, but the onus is on us to communicate them, and to communicate them all. Bach's music, born of church and cathedral, with the echoing chorus of choir, organ and congregation, is all-encompassing, not one lonely and isolated line of music, but a range and depth of voices living together, wrestling with and listening to each other. Bach's suites '*für* violoncello solo', for cello solo, demand an exploded interpretation of 'solo'. Performing the cello suites, I understand that my one cello occupying the stage carries a febrile, living weight of voices.

The art I practise is communication, and communication is not one-way. I communicate to audiences, with the voices and tides of the music. I listen and respond to my accompanists or sonata partners in the back-and-forth of musical conversation, contrapuntal or harmonic, contrasting or repetitive. I love to engage in an exhilarating call-and-response with an orchestra, throwing ideas between my individual cello and the mass of other instruments. When it's time for me to play a cadenza, I relish the momentary glare of that attention on me as an individual musician, but the moment is made meaningful by the poised, hushed waiting of the always anticipated orchestra.

All these insights grew out of my experiences with chamber music, which includes playing sonatas. Learning how to play chamber, as we call it, has informed my whole musical life. But it's not just my music-making that has been enriched by chamber music: in fact, it has infused, like a seeping, present ghost, a vast quantity of the music I've played and listened to. 'Chamber' is the intimate quality of listening and speaking to the voices close by. Chamber music is a conversation in a room, not an egotistical declaration in a concert hall. Yet the art of chamber is implied and alive in almost every iteration on the big stage. And any soloist who cannot play or doesn't understand chamber music risks missing the power and beauty of sonata and concerto music, and the significance of communicating and listening to others.

Originating from approximately the end of the eighteenth century, chamber music is traditionally music to be played in a chamber, or a room of a great house or palace. It is the music of salons and soirées, the smaller and more private social gatherings rather than the grand pomp and volume of opera houses or concert halls. And, for me, it is music between friends, rich with the banter and contest, the taking-turns and theme-sharing, of those who know or are getting to know each other well. I often get together with friends and siblings to sight-read or revisit new and long-beloved chamber pieces, be they for string quartet, piano quintet, multi-instrument ensembles, duets or sonatas. Chamber music sharpens my musical alertness, polishes my listening skills, and enlivens my ability to retort, to be heard, to join in. It's also extraordinary fun.

I was not born into the traditional background of a chamber musician. Our shelves weren't groaning with the stacked manuscripts of classical ensembles, and we certainly didn't have a grand, spacious, high-ceilinged drawing room with grand piano and ornate music stands. What we did have was a constant, energetic, imaginative and free world of conversation, the physical interaction of young, spirited children and a strong sense of play. And because of this, it feels as though the essence of chamber music was always there from the beginning, and a very natural part of my childhood.

As a gang of brothers and sisters, we were constantly enacting the spirit of chamber music. Before I opened my eyes in the morning, I was listening to conversation around me. Often, a brother or sister would bounce on my bed, or a soft ball or pillow would hit me in the face. I would be goaded until I toppled on to the floor and took up the chase. We were always creating something together in a world whose boundaries were each other's ideas. I remember the excitement of waking up to see the half-constructed village or house laid out in all its promise of cardboard, torn fabric pieces, glue, sellotape and paint. I remember the intake of breath before we pushed the domino-effect Jenga pieces into a long, curling snake of clattering wood along the entire length of the hallway, after my long-suffering mother had spent two days tiptoeing around it with the laundry baskets. We argued, long and passionately, over our dance moves for the loud and somersaulting shows we put on, and painted giant pictures on curling paper over tables and floor. The board games were tireless, with rules ever more complicated and contested, and sport or den-building or bow-and-arrow-making in the garden were all an extension of competitive discussion and debate. Our teasing of each other would develop into in-jokes that lasted for years. Nicknames would stick, themes and stories be repeated, tricks and ideas expanded or exaggerated. The aim was to make each other laugh – and to make our parents laugh – a feat we energetically competed to achieve. Creativity meant taking imaginative leaps and making risky suggestions that would either be vividly praised and embraced, or loudly rejected. The exciting dance move, the daring kick of the ball or sweep of the bat, the clever move in a game or brilliant gesture as you crashed downstairs on a cushion: all this was the essence of chamber music. The next line in an improvised rap, the funny anecdote, the cheekiest joke – this was all the essence of chamber music. And the gossip, rule-breaking and secrets of sibling life: all this was chamber music.

I have started with the feelings rather than the technical skill of chamber music because that's where the energy and the meaning begin. Encouraging children's imagination and sense of fun, as well as intimate connection with others, is the wellspring of musical generosity and communication. The joy of chamber music is the ability to test yourself against others, to be inspired by others, to push yourself technically and creatively into the arena, and it became as natural to me as breathing.

We began exploring group music through the Music for Everyone charity in Nottingham which ran courses for children's choir singing. Our mum was very keen that we should sing in choirs, and the vocal courses spanned two or three intensive weekends of group tuition with other Nottingham children, culminating in a big concert at Nottingham's Albert Hall. This allowed us to learn harmony and music-making with others before we began learning instruments, at least string instruments. We were all very young – I must have been three or four years old – and we were all excited to be taking part in this adventure.

We were given a cassette tape to play in our battered seven-seater. My parents would blast out the songs we had to learn on whatever trip we were going on. The best journeys were the three-hour car drives to visit Mama (our Welsh grandmother) in South Wales, or the similarly long trip to South London to visit our Antiguan grandparents. We would sing the songs in our best voices over and over again for as long as we could. At home, we carried on. I remember singing the songs for *Cats* and various other musicals that I never saw onstage. I loved learning the words and tunes to sing with Isata and Braimah. Even before I was old enough to join the first choir course they took part in, I learnt the songs anyway.

Since we started learning musical instruments, that knowledge of song has remained incredibly important. I consciously strive to sing through the cello. For someone like me who found expression through formal speech almost impossible as a child, the cello carried and held what I wanted to say. Where my public-speaking voice clogged up in my head, I found the cello took the shape and colour of what I felt and pulled it, burnished, cogent and full, into the room. Football in the playground and in the team had become an important thread of communication between me and the other boys at school, and music was giving me the same shining chance to share, with vigour and without obstruction, the feelings I kept inside.

When I look back, it seems like a natural and seamless move between childhood games, singing, cello and chamber, and I've retained those musical pathways, realizing more consciously why and how music is a living, live, changing and present phenomenon. But chamber music is also a discipline, and I understand that two things were happening concurrently through my childhood. While the choir courses were social, exciting and fun, they also required practice, learning lyrics, and perfecting pitch. We began learning instruments, beginning with piano, then stringed instruments, and we quickly understood the relationship between technique, sound and accuracy. Put simply, the techniques of fingering, posture and shaping, touch and phrasing, are indistinguishable from the music and have to be embedded and intrinsic to it. To play that phrase or thought or page, the technique is taken as read. But, in the first instance, it has to be taught and learnt.

Technique, tuning, getting better at solo playing for ourselves and by ourselves (or, often, with a teacher or parent) was important, but so too was it with accompaniment. A basic teaching (or parenting) trick was to play the bass or treble line on the keyboard an octave higher or lower while I stumbled or flowed through a piece. Equally, my cello teachers at various stages (Sarah Huson or Ben Davies) would play a harmony on their cellos as I played in lessons. This is incredibly useful for pitch and rhythm training, and wonderfully encouraging and uplifting for children. It made me feel as though I was really playing music.

Outside this framework of formal learning, we as siblings would mimic each other's pieces on our own instruments, or provide improvised harmony and counterbalance, coming into each other's practice spaces to join in, or echo each other's music from another room. Our solo practice would inevitably expand into duet-playing, or trio renditions, or full family ensembles as we wandered with our cellos, violins, viola into the hallway and pulled the door ajar to where the upright piano was pushed against the wall in the 'piano room'. Or, we would squeeze into the room and add one sibling after another on to the crowded rug, experimenting with a piece of music that belonged to one of our formal lessons. The game was to tease out or embellish the bass or treble sections, add harmony, modulations, or just volume to a piano, cello or violin piece that caught our imagination as a group. There are many pieces we learnt as children that exist between us in extended and enriched forms, developed to fill a room or a house of excited children set free with the rules.

Because, in the first instance, the rules mattered. This was mirrored in the games we played together. Without the rules, the games made no sense. We all had to operate within a framework we agreed to follow without dispute (although there was always a lot of loud discussion leading up to this) and whether they were games of imagination where no one really won, or sporting games – where winning was the point, even though the matches were on permanent repetition – rules and the skills that flourished within the rules were part of the joy. So it was with chamber music. We delighted in learning the art of it all and we wanted to get better at it.

Nothing can be broken, manipulated, re-formed and experimented with without first being learnt. Or perhaps it works both ways. We also began with improvisation before we embarked on the strict art of learning classical chamber pieces. And that spectrum of inventing, improvising, interpreting freely or accurately was explored in both directions for the years we were growing up.

We began with simple chamber pieces, or parts of works, like Haydn's 'Gypsy Rondo' from Piano Trio No. 39 in G, and Mozart's 'easy' trios for two violins and cello, or Frank Bridge's piano trios. We were introduced to these pieces by teachers or at music festivals, or on children's chamber music courses which our parents had found out about. The peer group we had at the Primary and Junior Royal Academy opened up a world of music which we could play together, and our parents were always having conversations with the teachers and with other parents to find out things they had had no idea about before. We would try many different classical duets, from Beethoven's and Mozart's piano duets, to Johan Halvorsen's virtuosic transcription of Handel's 'Passacaglia', arranged for violin and cello. We loved Bartók's duos for two violins, or violin and cello, and many arrangements of pieces for 'weddings', which simplified choral or orchestral repertoire – or popular tunes – into written parts for string quartet. Often, we would get excited about pieces that were still too advanced for us to play, but that we had witnessed older children playing, or watched famous musicians perform on YouTube. We would try them anyway, giddy with the fantasy that we were performing in public venues to hushed audiences, thrilled with the music we were delivering together. That mixture of heady role play, of grappling with music and ideas that are yet too difficult, in an environment where everyone celebrates the noise for what it is – communal joy – is an essential element of complex and curious musicianship.

I remember Isata, Braimah and I insisting we could play Shostakovich's Piano Trio No. 2, especially the fourth movement, which we thought – at the ages of nine, ten and twelve – could have been written for us. It was intricate, complicated, wild and precise, like a storm full of biting humour, caged in the music. We were all utterly entranced by it and launched into it with regular ferocity for years until we really could play it on the public stage. What we discovered, and kept discovering, was that the process of mastering something is as endless and open-ended as relationships, experience and collective memories. We are always constrained by the limits of our skills, our preferences and our knowledge, but musical understanding lives and grows in the boundless exchange of inspiration with others.

We moved from and between duets and trios, quartets, quintets, sextets and septets with different combinations of instruments, sometimes improvised or copied from what we had heard on the radio or CDs, sometimes and increasingly from written chamber parts. We played music together just as we played together as brothers and sisters. It was joyful, collegiate and challenging. And then, we were lucky enough to be *taught*. Our parents recognized that having lessons on our separate instruments, while vital, wasn't enough. They asked our string teachers, first, to give us duet and trio lessons, and I remember Sarah Huson and Siân Evans coming to the house to help us play the first movement of Mendelssohn's piano trio when we were advanced enough to play the notes but needed to understand the extra, larger 'meta' space where the music lived beyond and between us. This was an art form that relied on more than banter and competitive conversation, that was a greater creation needing a tender reverence and intensity of listening which we had to practise.

A major moment in my life was auditioning for the Primary department of the Royal Academy of Music in London. The Primary and Junior Academy have become part of the fabric of my childhood and life as a musician. But I don't want to forget what a conscious and decided leap it was to get there. Isata auditioned when she had just turned ten years old and it was her determination to go that started a family tradition. My parents had never heard of this Saturday school for under-eighteens and when Isata mentioned it at the age of nine, having heard about it in a casual conversation, they looked it up. My mother was immediately worried as it relied on competitive national auditions, had limited places, and was very difficult to get into. Isata also played piano, and piano and strings were – and are – hotly competitive instruments. My dad decided it was merely a matter of practice – albeit a lot of practice – and for a year, Isata seemed to be working incredibly hard. We watched and were fascinated by this, and intrigued by her longing, her drive and the emotional effort it all seemed to be exacting from her.

After the audition, which was in London and seemed to last a whole day, we all waited nervously to see what the outcome was. I was seven years old and had been playing the cello for only half a year, but I already knew that this was my instrument. When Isata's letter arrived, telling my parents she had been offered a place for the following September, there was an explosion of excitement that changed the air in the house. If this was possible, then so was so much more. From that point, the level of practice, and what that practice meant, seemed to reach a higher level. Isata began travelling to London with either or both parents every Saturday and suddenly we were all focused on what instrument-learning meant at a national level. Isata and then the rest of us in the years to come (I was nine years old when I auditioned) were set in the midst of those children who were preparing to enter the conservatoires, the orchestras, the international competitions and music profession of the future. From that moment, everything changed.

Joining the Primary Royal Academy and being taught to play chamber music with children outside the family was a revelation for me, as well as the string chamber group run by Sarah and Siân, and the residential chamber courses we attended. I then had to collaborate with personalities I did not know intimately, could not second-guess, and who had skills and musical intuition in areas and moments that were a complete surprise to me. Not knowing what was going to happen before it did was a great lesson in thinking on my feet. As siblings, we always tried to surprise each other, trip each other up in ways that would make us alert and creative. In these new ensembles, the very rules had to be searched for and understood again, with a new web of musical etiquette which, while I missed the shortcuts, was challenging and refreshing, sending me along unpredictable paths. I found I had to prove myself anew and over again. Musical alertness here also meant a keen sense of danger, and nothing could be taken for granted.

We all found ourselves thrown into the arena of

proving ourselves, keeping up, comparing ourselves to the musical fluency of others. The Primary and Junior Academy of Music, and the chamber music courses we attended, thrust us into the wider world of instrumental music where individual musical personality mattered, but only in the heated, testing, supportive exchange of a team dedicated to something bigger and brighter than each other. Isata, Braimah and I also auditioned for the National Youth Chamber Orchestra, run by David and Gill Johnston, and loved the larger orchestral sound we could be part of, encompassing all the instruments of the orchestra, yet retaining the sense of intimacy and self-recognition we had grown to rely on. The standard was very high and we were challenged and stretched, while being thrown into a collective of children of which we began to see ourselves as members – even though our weekday and school lives might have been a class apart.

Chamber music is a very human, social way of making music in a team, relying on trust and the ability to exchange ideas, to disagree and to compromise, to respond and to cooperate. It taught me huge respect for others and a realization that musical ego, while necessary to be heard and counted, needs limits.

I will never forget my first encounter with the London Haydn Quartet, through MusicWorks, the chamber course we attended every summer from our mid-teens to the end of school. MusicWorks taught me the practical meaning of the music theory I had been learning in my grade exams and at Junior Royal Academy. The emphasis on musical harmony and structure made vivid, visceral sense to me through the depth and wealth of chamber music we played for several summers at Music-Works. The connection between music theory and music practice dawned on me, marvellously, through playing chamber music.

Hearing the Haydn Quartet play live in concerts and listening to their recordings, I felt a drama and an awe that almost drowned me. The members of the string quartet – changed in different recordings but consistently including one of its founding members, Catherine Manson – were so in tune with each other that individuality should have been sacrificed to a stronger beast, and yet it lived as though hypnotized in an excruciating depth of concentration I didn't want to break. Four voices became a body of conjoined meaning and emotion that couldn't have been achieved by one person and was astonishingly beautiful and painfully present. I knew, while my breath almost stopped, that here was music I couldn't emulate alone. Here was music for which cathedrals were built and its divinity existed in the generosity of its unlimited communality. I could hear each salient solo part, each breath-stroke note, yet what I ultimately heard were shared chords so blended and textual with voices they bristled with life. And I knew that chamber music was an art form I would always seek out.

*

Now, my life as an international soloist involves playing many solo cello recitals, or concertos (concerti) with orchestras where I am the soloist, and these concerts are vital for me. But every musician needs the opportunity to play music with their peers. Organizations like IMS Prussia Cove, Rosendal Chamber Music Festival and Highgate International Chamber Music Festival, for example, are so important for professional soloists to perform together. They are places where international professional musicians can meet to play for fun, and to learn from each other. The performances are serious and high-level, and the friendships made and kept are important. However, chamber music is not just about internationally celebrated musicians coming together. I have always played chamber music with siblings and close friends such as Harry Baker and Plínio Fernandes, for example, in concerts, living rooms, in recordings, on many stages and none. Chamber music, where we get to meet face-to-face, and hear, up close, the vibrancy and immediacy of our different musical personalities and ideas, keeps us connected, challenged, inspired and supported.

For pianists like my sisters, chamber is the bedrock of their playing. They say that the piano is often like a chamber group in itself and to understand the harmonic lines, the voices in the chords and the scope of the music demands a deep appreciation of how chamber music works. I've often acted as part of an audience for when two sisters practise piano concertos together. We have two pianos in the 'piano room' at home in Nottingham, and we've had this arrangement of one grand piano and an upright together for a number of years. One sister who is practising a concerto will play her solo part, with the other sister playing the piano reduction of the orchestra on the upright. When the grand piano we had was even worse than the upright, they were forced to switch that round! It's always like a double lesson in solo and chamber-playing, with the solo pianist's ego constantly upheld or challenged by the orchestral piano, and forced to battle for voice in the call-and-response, or the counter-unity of orchestra and soloist. Then comes the moment where the orchestra piano lays down the gauntlet in the ultimate challenge of the piano cadenza, where the piano soloist strikes out into the orchestra's waiting, heavy silence to play alone with the themes, phrases, melody and ideas of the whole ensemble. The cadenza becomes a rendition of the orchestra itself in that distilled, crystallized momentous spotlight of loneliness that nevertheless recalls the might of orchestral sound.

Another experience that lives with me is when three of my sisters (at the ages of twelve, fourteen and eighteen), played Bach's Toccata in F major, arranged for three pianos, as well as Mozart's Triple Concerto (No. 7) with Djanogly Community Orchestra at Trinity School in Nottingham. This was a feast of chamber music, where the cadenzas felt like chamber trio performance. Here was the dazzling repartee of three pianists waging war and peace with each other and it was amazing – and rare – to hear three grand pianos together like this. I witnessed a dance of intricate timing where all three had to remain alive to two other soloists as well as being vigilant to a whole orchestra, and I loved the playing out of this live tightrope of exposure and togetherness, culminating in a triumphant, chordal cadence.

Since then, I have played and toured Beethoven's Triple Concerto with Isata and Braimah, and performed and recorded it with Nicola Benedetti and Ben Grosvenor on Decca Classics. The 'Beethoven Triple' has three soloists in front of the orchestra – piano, violin and cello – and playing this is very much a meeting between piano trio performance and concerto playing. It's brilliantly a solo concerto and a chamber trio and moves restlessly between the two (related) forms of music.

For me, the path still stretches from those moments as a child or young teenager when I was exposed to chamber music to now, where I am a concert soloist. What it means and how it feels has stayed with me from those days of dreaming and experimenting in our hallway all the way to the sold-out Festival Hall concert in London where I played with Nicola and Ben, two renowned international soloists.

When I remember our first public performance of chamber music as a very young sibling piano trio, I can see how chamber music took me to television appearances, to winning BBC Young Musician at the age of sixteen, and to playing at a globally screened royal wedding in the heart of Windsor. The art of chamber music took me to my performances at the BAFTAs and to concert halls around the world. Chamber music helped to form me into the musician I am today, which is bigger and more significant than the nuggets of newsworthy achievements along the way. My relationship with my brother and my five sisters, formed out of music and play, has been burnished by the years of playing music together, practising and rehearsing together, and learning to speak and play the turbulent, lively language of the brilliant, demanding, extraordinary chamber music we have discovered, and written or arranged, ourselves. What chamber music has done is keep our family close.

3. Education and Opportunity

When I was three years old, my parents took me and my siblings to a village near Nottingham where we visited a shop full of pianos. I'm not sure if this is an authentic memory or a reconstruction in my mind because I seem to have always lived with a piano nearby. But the upright Yamaha piano we bought that day would be the beginning of something endless, and endlessly growing, for all of us. The piano appeared in our house and was placed in what was then the 'dining room' but immediately became and remained the 'piano room'. Isata, as the eldest, began learning first, and I was fascinated. It is only a small upright piano, but to me then it was huge, humming, almost alive in its great wooden skin. My sister was able to make this clanging, echoing, percussive creature sing to her with the music we heard on the radio, or on CDs. The piano room became a place of pilgrimage where the door stayed open for us to hear what Isata was playing, directly through her own body, while the piano translated, reordered and magnified her voice. Every day, I would lean or stand against the piano while Isata played. Because we were all so close as children, Isata simply accepted me crawling on the floor by the pedals or pushing a toy car over floorboards radiating with piano vibrations while she practised.

I have been lucky in so many ways. My family surrounded me with music and my elder brother and sister showed me how far I could go as I watched them forging the road. Lessons were learnt and mistakes made by my siblings – and me – from which I could learn first-hand. I was ushered, very naturally, into the wonder and delight of the world of music. But perhaps more significant than any of this is the fact that music was something in which I was *educated*.

From a very young age, my introduction to music was holistic. Music entered my imagination, my mind and my body. I was drawn into listening to recordings and to the bustle of live music being played – and played with – in my own home. Music was sublime and perfect and direct. It was also malleable, difficult, built on experiment, practice, mistakes and changing ideas. It was something to create, wrestle with, be challenged by and be reinterpreted in the restless, energetic, growing, social intelligence of childhood, demanding effort and optimism.

I was lucky. At the age of five, I went to my brother's and sister's state school, Walter Halls Primary, within Nottingham city, where, under the headship of Peter Strauss, music ranked equally with maths, English, history, science, art and sport. I learnt to transfer the idea of practice, effort and wonder, to and between all subjects, an approach that was encouraged through conversations and examples from my parents. Maths fascinated me with its patterns of logic and possibility. Numbers, equations and sums were not fixed but open-ended in combination and method. Simple elements combined into intricate, surprising results. Learning to read involved the alignment of letters to sound, and then words and sentences. A story was bigger than the hard nuggets of stilted letters, and the leap to rhythm, narrative and meaning was almost a matter of blind faith. History was an uncovering of what had been, but was fraught with contrasting points of view and stimulated the need to make comparisons, reflect on change and develop empathy. Science was the play between hard facts and their demonstration in the world, as well as imaginative theories of what was unseen or dimly, incredibly fathomable. Art demanded the free play of thought, interpretation, accuracy and beauty, and sport let free my physical drive and passion, pitting strength and wits against others, and honing attention to strategy, prediction and immediacy. All demanded technique. All demanded practice. All resulted in something greater and more beautiful than their first, raw and individual elements.

I didn't realize then that education was a site of fervent disagreement, or that children were subject to policy decisions and curriculum changes that could impact so much of our lives. I am continually surprised now when anyone accepts the hard walls built between creativity and science, or between the arts and maths as though they are self-evident, rather than spurious and political.

Music infused the time we all came together as a class or as a school. We were a mixed collection of city children, predominantly working-class with a minority of middle-class families and those who were involved in the arts, ethnically diverse and with a range of languages. Many children had mixed heritage and several came from all parts of the world. We were told to file into assembly in an orderly manner while music surrounded us from a speaker as we walked in lines to sit cross-legged on the floor.

I remember filing in to the warm arpeggios and cadences of Yo-Yo Ma's Bach cello suites, responding to the calm concentration that washed over me. We were all listening, as though our minds were taken elsewhere while still being embedded in the present. The separate yet blended notes and sequences of the cello were replaced by the depth of an orchestra of instruments in Dvořák's 'New World' Symphony, taking us through an exploration of folk music and classical form. We entered this realm of new and jostling voices with clear signposts. A poster would be pinned to the wall when we filed in, giving the title of the piece, the composer and performer, and in the wonderment of this expedition through new landscapes, we were allowed to know and therefore own what we heard. We absorbed the hymns we sang in assembly and looked forward to their familiar repetition. The school choir introduced singing in harmony, and from the age of eight we could begin to learn an instrument.

Playing together as a class or in groups within the classroom was the first step to really understanding the role of playing with others. I was already having individual piano and cello lessons outside school, but I valued this time of musical collaboration with my school friends. We played simple jazz together, instructed to take it in turns in a build-up of musical call-and-response. I played trombone and also trumpet, enrolling in the guitar group as well as in the choir. The school's regular Music Nights, with parents, friends and family in the audience, featured the brass and woodwind groups taught as part of the curriculum, the choir, guitar group, violin group, recorders, drumming and any individual or duo contributions volunteered by the children themselves. The excitement of those nights was intoxicating. The preparation was part of school life, the partnerships with each other important, and we learnt to see, in greater fullness and clarity, who we were and who we could be.

It was on one of these music nights that I gave a performance of a cello piece, accompanied by my sister Isata on the old school upright piano, driving utter commitment into the Romantic classical piece I had learnt, W. H. Squire's rousing *Tarantella*. This virtuosic cello piece shows off so much of what the cello can do – impressive

fast passages, flowing, expansive phrases and a breathtaking, exciting ending. The piano part relies on rippling
notes and blazing chords, and even though we were two
young children we took control of the performance and
made it our own. The fact that we were both having
advanced one-to-one instrument lessons outside school
is important. I was about eight years old, and Isata had
just turned eleven. By then, Isata had already gained
the highest marks in the UK for Grades 7 and 8 piano
with two Gold Awards from the Associated Board of
the Royal Schools of Music, ABRSM, and I had passed
Grade 7 cello with Distinction. This was a moment of
bringing our extracurricular education and intense hard
work into a school that cared. It mattered to us that who
we were outside school could be visible inside. It mattered that our lives in school and with our friends didn't
exist in a world apart from our lives in music.

There was a hushed silence in the room as we played.
I looked hard at everyone, needing the attention of each
person in the audience while submerged in the necessity of the rhythm and pace of the piece, locked in an
intense symbiosis of piano and cello. At the end, the
room erupted with applause.

There have been many performances – recitals, concertos, large and smaller crowds, places and contexts – but
this moment stands out as a turning point. I was given,
in one place, a convergence of myself as schoolchild,
friend, pupil, son and brother. And in this place, in my

school, I was given the identity of a musician. For a child, the importance of performing to and receiving attention from those around them is paramount. School is central to the community that children inhabit, and the school environment has a major impact on children's sense of self-worth. My cello lessons took place outside school, but because music was respected and taught within school, I could enter with my cello and have the chance to be myself.

Schools can light the flame of learning music, and provide the context to express it. Collaborative musical education is vital and, if provided with enthusiasm and skill, has an intense impact on children's lives. Music is something to be learnt and shared with others, and taking ownership of learning happens when a child can demonstrate their own place within it.

The moment of performance is powerful. When I played *Tarantella* to my school community I was the subject of my own destiny. For the duration of the piece, I was noticed and appreciated, and in this, the effort of learning had its reward. Schools take many hours of a child's life every day and have to be responsible for a large part of children's well-being, confidence and sense of self. Being able to join in, to learn or show off a skill set that delights, moves and impresses others, and demands a level of application and responsibility – this was allowed to be central to my experience of school.

Almost all my classmates were present at Music Night

and the school hall was filled with primary school children ready to demonstrate musical skills they had practised at home, or with their friends. It was a night of group and solo singing, guitars, recorders, drums, brass and wood-wind. There was dancing and rap, musical theatre and the school choir. The vast majority of children didn't have music tuition outside school, but some took lessons within school time from visiting music teachers. Some took dance or singing lessons out of school hours, but most just wanted to take part, and felt they could. Talent was applauded, but so was the sheer energy and courage of performing, and I learnt then that connecting with an audience is not solely about talent. What children have to offer and gain is far greater than only a God-given ability.

There was one particular pupil at my school who I'd noticed had been somewhat dismissed, not cruelly but with a sort of uninterest, as someone who wasn't very good at school. And then, one year, they were given an opportunity to sing in a school performance. I hardly thought about it, and if I did, I probably assumed that the teachers were being kind to them, or to their parents, by giving them a turn at being the star, even only for five minutes. I do remember worrying that it might go the other way: that their behaviour, which was often 'chal-lenging', might ruin their moment in the spotlight. But oh, how wrong I was! On the night, the performance was going well, or at least as well as a primary school perform-ance can, with anything that went wrong being greeted with indulgent laughter, and a general air of excitement and anticipation growing with each scene. Then, it was time for the big solo and this pupil, from whom no one expected anything, came up on to the stage. The music from the accompanying guitar and drum section started up and we waited, in nervous anticipation, for it to be over. Would they start acting up as usual and mess up their moment? Up until this point, the only attention they ever got was negative, and I was worried that they wouldn't be able to resist another fight with the world. I will never forget what actually happened. Out of this pupil's mouth and body came a voice so clear and direct, so tuneful and expressive, that I stopped fidgeting and sank into the charmed silence that had suddenly filled the hall. Everyone sat or stood and looked at this small pupil, who had always been at the centre of trouble, and heard something beautiful. Their face was transformed by a sincerity I didn't know was there and the song they sang changed the atmosphere in the room. We were all stunned. After that, their status in the school changed and the settled picture of them that I held in my head blurred and shifted. I hadn't expected to be moved. I hadn't known who they were until they started to sing.

So what happens when music is drained out of the classroom, the assembly hall, the special or after-school event, the small groups, the individual instruction? What happens if children are given music at primary school level and then enter a musical wasteland at secondary school? What happens if children are not given any musical education at all?

State education is built around an understanding of what are deemed to be 'core' subjects, the essential learning that all children cannot be without and to which other subjects should be secondary. What are called worthy subjects in the school curriculum have been driven by the promotion of STEM which calculates the crucial subjects that children need. Neither thread of these governing directives in state school education has time for music.

'Core' subjects are English, Maths and Science. 'STEM' subjects elbow English out of the pantheon of worth to allow room instead for only science, technology, engineering and maths. Any subjects brushed by the tinge of a leaning to the arts no longer get a mention.

Of course, I respect the value of these core or STEM subjects. Maths, science, technology and engineering are fascinating and valuable pursuits, with technology and engineering built on the foundation of science and maths. But if we stop there, and concentrate only on developing this knowledge and intelligence, what do we lose both now and in the future?

There are two aspects that fuel the argument. One is that what makes children clever and builds better brains are the fact-based, evidence-heavy, solid bricks of serious, mathematical study. The idea is that exam outcomes are regularly quantifiable and easily assessed. Children are given weighty, useful knowledge they can steadily accrue. Students are told repeatedly that the working world which awaits them after school overwhelmingly demands employees who understand the nuts and bolts of technology, business, finance and scientific progress.

The shadow-side of these arguments, the belief that lies underneath, is that arts subjects educate children in ways that are non-essential. By teaching children to feel, imagine, be happy, express themselves and communicate, the idea is that real – essential – learning has been avoided. The creative and performing arts are seen as light, wishy-washy, unquantifiable pursuits that cannot be effectively marked and rely on subjectivity rather than the neutrality of objective judgement. In this argument, the world of work has no place for people who think in an undisciplined way, who have not toed the line within strict educational boundaries and who cannot obviously slide into the only viable jobs that exist – those in science, maths, banking, technology and business. Articles like, for example, the one written by Helena Pozniak for the *Telegraph* (29 November 2019): 'Work in STEM and the World is your Oyster', terrorize young people with questions like: 'How employable are you?' The list of top ten useful subjects for employability are all in science, engineering and business studies, and the article claims: 'Employment rates are higher for STEM graduates than all other graduates.' Yet, further down the article – away from its titles and subtitles – is the acknowledgement that creativity, communication skills and a grudging nod to the arts will always be vital, if hidden beneath the clarion call for STEM-only education. Professor Rebecca Shipley, a 'mathematician who now works in medical engineering' is quoted as saying: 'Some of the most exciting challenges require people from many different disciplines.'

Presented as 'common-sense' conclusions, the accepted dismissal of creative arts subjects lies almost undisturbed on the surface of public discussion and policy decisions. Musicians repeatedly find themselves pushed into defensive positions based on the 'truth' of these assumptions. My experience with music and the creative arts has no reflection in this parade of facts and my ability to be self-disciplined, to connect with and respond to others, and to think laterally, are all qualities developed through music. In addition, science, maths and engineering are subjects that also require creative thinking, invention and teamwork. Any business needs communication, self-expression and performance, and the world of work within a thriving economy includes the economic juggernaut of the music and creative arts industry. And it is certainly not true that the only viable jobs are in the science, technology and banking sectors, unless we need to unpick what we each mean by 'viable'.

A fascinating article in the *Times Education Supplement* (*TES* magazine, 16 August 2023) written by the president of the British Science Association, Dr Anne-Marie

Imafidon, in collaboration with the president, Professor Julia Black, of the British Academy ('the UK's national body for the humanities and social sciences') takes issue with the educational dichotomy between the sciences and the arts. Many of the ideas supporting the need for this rift are based on false presumptions that need to be carefully dismantled. They identify a gulf between 'Shape' (social sciences, humanities and the arts for people and the economy) and 'Stem' (science, technology, engineering and maths). They argue that the long-standing emphasis by politicians to 'talk down the value of the arts and humanities' has resulted in an 'imbalance', both in education and in the resulting workforce.

Arguing against a 'narrative that pits some subjects against others', and promoting 'Connected Knowledge', or collaboration between the sciences and the arts, their vision is a workforce that can address the challenges of AI, climate change, 'scientific, technical and data analysis', cultural, linguistic and historical understanding between societies, health and the quality of life by combining skills from both 'sides'. If we don't restructure education policies to 'share and celebrate' knowledge between the arts and sciences, the losses will affect future generations: 'The reductive approach to learning leads to tunnel vision in the way we structure the economy, design industrial strategies and think about big societal challenges.'

This viewpoint is amply backed up by the Higher

Education Policy Institute report (HEPI Report 159: 'The Humanities in the UK Today: What's Going On?' 2023) which quotes 'one employer of a large tech corporation' as saying: 'The way I view it is, if you're going into more STEM-based or more business-focused degrees, longer term, you still need a foundation in the Humanities; you need to have an understanding of language and communication and philosophy in order to do those other things.'

Of course, we have to be careful not to reduce the arts to the service of a 'more important' scientific world. The creative arts are more than just transferable skills and can and should, like science and maths, be an end in themselves.

Perhaps there are political and social reasons why state schools are placed in this ever more rigid dichotomy between arts and sciences, where each side is given undoubted and uncontested characteristics and assessed accordingly. I never experienced this watershed between maths and music, or between science and literature, for example, on which recent theories of education insist.[1] If we accept this argument, we agree that maths, science and technology do not require imagination, lateral thinking, or creative intelligence, which is clearly untrue. To do well in business, sales or marketing certainly needs a deep understanding of people, and the skills of self-presentation or 'telling the story' really do matter beyond arts institutions. The ability to learn languages – whether of other countries or of different kinds of texts – is crucial in the world of banking and artificial intelligence. The training to read between the lines, to understand the culture, ideas and social framework of dramatic or narrative literature, or music, or art has evident relevance in the world of profit and loss, of international deals, or politics. And the confidence to create something individual, revolutionary or unique, or to respond in new ways to old or entrenched ideas, or simply to identify with emotion, beauty or pain, are skills much needed in the workforce. And if we need them in the workforce, we need them in our national culture too.

What happens when we refuse to include these skills in our majority state school population and thereby devalue artistic expression and creative output? If we are told, exclusively, what facts are, and what truth is, how do we learn to think analytically and creatively about anything?

The world of work is defined by what we educate children to do and how. There's no reason to doubt the power and relevance of the creative industries. During the Covid pandemic, people longed for live music, theatre and ballet. They could no longer buy tickets for shows that had been closed down, and concerts that had been cancelled. The demand for online or televised performances rapidly increased and the huge losses in the music industry contributed to serious, long-term effects on the economy.

The extent to which the world of work includes the much-wanted and much-loved performing arts is tied, not just to how much financial support the sector receives, but to its social and cultural value. If we strip music from schooling, we enter a process of de-education, of un-skilling the next generation of potential artists and musicians, and telling them that music is frivolous and unimportant. By extension, we tell them (and their parents) that, if they attempt to pursue these subjects, they will also become frivolous and unimportant.

The idea that music is an extracurricular activity is responsible for, or a product of, the funding squeeze, or complete lack of funding in schools. It has always been recognized as a serious subject to be studied at elite universities, who require applicants to have studied sufficiently 'academic' subjects at A level and recognize music as one of these, yet the budget of political will is lagging behind. What will happen, and is already happening, is not so much that music and the performing arts will disappear, because they are desired by a population that needs cultural activities and music as part of being human. The result is actually that the music and arts industry ends up being *practised only* by those groups in society that are lucky enough to be offered an education in the arts, an education whose value is increasingly contested and increasingly expensive. Lack of arts education leads to a reduction in the diversity of arts production and consumption. The energy and vitality of artistic output and of audiences can only dampen and shrink in an enforced monoculture.

In effect we have a two-tier education system in the UK, and its result is that we are educating our children differently from each other, along lines of disadvantage and plenty. Private schools offer prestigious music scholarships for skilled young musicians, and their music facilities are often state-of-the-art. For example, Eton College's website boasts of an astonishing offering of 'two concert halls, a recording studio, three music technology suites, drum suites, a music library, and a large number of teaching and practice rooms'. They also advertise music scholarships: 'Each year, around 27 boys from a wide variety of backgrounds arrive at Eton as part of our Music Award programme, receiving specialist support to develop their musical talents.' Similarly, on their website, Winchester College does not shy away from music as a valid, worthy, career aspiration: 'Music Awards are available to any candidate who shows exceptional musical talent. Many former pupils have highly successful careers as performers, conductors and composers'. And at Marlborough College, the website acknowledges and encourages music as a significant career possibility: 'Where applicable, individual learning programmes are designed to meet the demands and needs of those wishing to study music at conservatoire or university following Marlborough.'

To be educated in music within these schools, or

outside, requires money, or class status, or luck. It also requires desire, belief and an appreciation of the importance of music. And all this comes hand-in-hand with education and access.

The perceived elitism of classical music arises from precisely this situation within music education and state schooling. If state school children do not have access to learning a musical instrument, or to hearing certain kinds of music, whether on recordings or in live concerts, we cement their perception that classical music is elitist. Then, if we look at the audiences in concert halls, or take one glance at the musicians onstage, or view the concert planners, artists' managers and recording companies behind them, we will only see wealth, or private education, or class uniformity, or luck. And because of both the demographics and cultural ideas of education and success, fostered within schooling, there will be – and is – very little ethnic diversity. 'High' culture ends up talking to only one group of people, with shared ideas and ideals, and with limited experiences and backgrounds. The boundaries between classical and non-classical music become stultifying and the barriers rigid and insuperable. In this situation, myths abound about worth or cultural value. Disadvantaged and non-White populations are encouraged to think that classical music is not 'for' them, that it is practised and listened to in spaces both revered and impenetrable. Collaboration between genres of music, and the growth, change, energy and continuation of classical music, become threatened. The loss to all music in these spiralling echo-chambers is devastating.

I am describing the probable result of a continuing status quo, and projecting into a future determined by educational directives. We are already there, in many ways, but we are also not there yet. Classical music is not elitist and I enjoy a flourishing, exciting and incredibly busy career playing with extraordinary musicians and to enthusiastic and engaged audiences all over the world. The curiosity and excitement are there, and I see the vast possibilities in an emerging new generation of children and teenagers. But I also feel the gap between the world of music and creativity I experience and the tales being told to so many schools and by so many legislators. If we are to turn the wheel the other way, we need to tackle the assumption that the world of work beyond school is one of computable production where jobs are reduced to saleable components and education itself is reduced to jobs. What is the purpose of education and what is the world of work and employment? The argument is not already won and the answers do not all come from one place. Humans cannot live on bread alone. Human intelligence is not artificial intelligence.

Because of my combination of school and family background, I had the opportunity to become cultur-ally bilingual. My primary and secondary schools were in geographical areas of disadvantage, with an ethnically mixed intake and large class sizes. In addition, because I came from a Black family, I was statistically very unlikely to become a classical musician.[2] Yet I have been lucky enough to achieve this.[3]

My parents and grandparents had access, of varying degrees, to school music education, and the particular schools I went to embraced and encouraged music as their ideological bedrock. I was also lucky with timing. Before I left school in 2017, there was still a lot of freedom for headteachers and leadership teams to fore-ground music and to spend their budget more freely. Decision-making was more centred in the individual school, and general funding more generous. Moving music provision in England from 2011 outside schools to be centred in the Music Hubs – departments that employ and administer music teachers, expertise and equipment needed for music education, funded by the Arts Council England – has made music a non-statutory choice for those responsible for a dwindling school budget. Reducing the funding to Hubs and making them responsible for persuading school leaders to take on their services has radically impacted the kind of school music experience I was so lucky to enjoy. As Deborah Annetts of the Independent Society of Musicians has stated, 'Funding for Hubs hasn't increased since 2016 or kept up with inflation, despite an increase in the number of pupils in our schools'.[4] In this way, the conditions in state schools have steadily declined, and music is being shunted out under a more centralized, dictatorial and reduced budget.

My secondary school, Trinity Catholic School, was extraordinary for a state secondary. When I entered as an eleven-year-old, thrilled to finally wear the same blazer and tie as my sister and brother, I was anticipating the orchestra I would join, the music groups I could be a part of, and the huge school concerts in which I could play. I would be part of the orchestra for the whole school show, and I was determined to join the boys' choir. There is a photo of me on my first day, standing next to my brother in our school uniforms, me looking very small and very excited, and both of us brimming with pride.

I've often wondered why schools that have outstanding academic results, happy and well-behaved pupils, a great sense of belonging and social cohesion, are not emulated by other schools or city councils. Music was introduced to Trinity by an earlier headteacher, Mr Bonner, when it was seen as a failing school. He ordered a big load of cheap violins and recorders, because they were affordable, and made it mandatory for every pupil who entered the school to learn how to play them. Those who were already very proficient on an instrument could use these group lessons to go into vacant music rooms to practise. Very quickly, the school was judged Outstanding by Ofsted[5] and remained a beacon school for years, because the headteachers, Mr Bonner, Mr McKeever and Mr Dexter were determined to saturate Trinity with music and thereby transform the collective ethos.

I already had Grade 8 on the cello, which is the final grade level for instrumentalists and has traditionally been the standard expected from the eighteen-year-old school leavers who are advanced in music and may wish to study further at university level. In their guidance for prospective pupils, specialist music schools advise those who are considered musically gifted to aim for Grade 8 standard by the age of thirteen. When I achieved Grade 8 with Distinction with ABRSM at the age of nine, it reassured my parents that music was something I could pursue seriously, and gaining the highest marks for Grade 8 cello in the UK that year was also a validation for them that what I loved and wanted to do was a realistic choice.

I had begun my stringed instrument-learning on the violin at the age of five. But this had not gone well. I remember my frustration that my brother, seventeen months my senior, was more advanced than me, and that he could play the violin with ease. His sound and confidence were a rebuke to my awkward grappling with shoulder, chin and bow, and I was in no mood to listen to my mother's painstaking instructions. Both Isata and Braimah played violin as well as piano, and they were more advanced than me on both. Being the third child made me determined to find my own place and my own

voice. This was similar to my desperation to be a con-
tender when I played football or cricket with Braimah,
Isata and Dad, or chess and Monopoly. It was always
me who raged, boiling over with the ferocious effort of
keeping up, annoyed by being smaller and less experienced than my elder siblings. It's a time in my childhood
that still amuses us all, but probably determined the path
I took in music, and my commitment to being heard.

I discovered the cello almost by chance, and it changed
my life. Isata and Braimah were taking part in a performance in Nottingham with Stringwise. Run by Music for
Everyone, this was an initiative that provided courses
in string orchestral playing for children in Nottingham
at different levels of expertise. For several intensive
days spread over two or three weekends, children came
together to learn to play with others in a string orchestra of their own level, and to perform as part of their
orchestra groups in a massed concert on the final
Sunday. I was in the audience, six years old, sitting with
Mum, Dad and my three younger sisters. It was in Nottingham's Albert Hall, with its semicircular seating, and
we found ourselves just behind the cello section in the
group of the most advanced teenagers.

I was transfixed, and my parents tell me I have never
sat so still. In normal circumstances I was always fidgeting, and my primary school teachers would comment at
every parents' evening that I was incapable of sitting on

a chair, always bouncing on my knees or hopping about. The issue wasn't a lack of concentration, but rather a kind of excessive physicality. I wanted to run, climb (including bookcases, doors and walls), play football, wrestle in the hallway or do gymnastics with my brother. If I needed to read or write, I had to simultaneously allow the agitation to flow through my body and express what I was thinking through visible movement. My parents simply accepted this. They didn't disassociate different forms of energy, and if movement represented thought, or dreaming, or active problem-solving, that was fine.

But now, at the Stringwise concert, close to the cello section, my whole body was centred in an uncharacteristic calm and I was stricken with this sound I had entered for the first time. This live, in-person cello music was singing to me and I didn't want to move, or fidget or bounce. This was where I wanted to be and I needed to get closer. Straight after the concert, I began. My parents were distracted with praising Isata and Braimah and managing two little girls and a small baby, but I kept on, regardless. 'I want to play *that*. I want to play a *cello*. *When* can I learn the cello?'

My parents had decided and arranged with careful thought and planning that the three of us would play piano and violin. I had been bought a cheap, quarter-size violin and I inherited the sheet music and instruction of my elder siblings. Mum had taken lessons from scratch on the violin the year before, and in a year gained Grade

5 so she could help us with the rudiments before having to pay for a teacher. She saw the piano as the fundamental and basic instrument. Both of my parents were brought up with piano lessons. My Welsh grandmother was given piano lessons as a child because the instrument was well respected in her Baptist chapel upbringing. The piano, organ and singing were central to a society organized around community, religion and music, so my mother was also given this chance to learn. My father's mother played piano throughout her childhood in Antigua, one of twelve children in a family that also valued the piano. My father and his sister were expected to learn and practise diligently.

The violin was introduced through my own mother's unfulfilled childhood longing to play the violin, and also the fact that my Antiguan grandfather had learnt as a child and might have gone so much further if his parents could have afforded more lessons. Even though my parents' second instruments at school had been clarinet and cello, the violin was presented as the most practical and most prized of orchestral – and therefore social – instruments to play. On the one hand, for my mother, the violin held the most ethereal and elusively beautiful voice to unlock and master. And on the other hand, a family of several children naturally functions in regimented, streamlined ways. If every child learnt piano and violin, it was simply the most economical and efficient way of managing the challenges of myriad costs, the spiralling expense of music books and of growing children needing new and bigger violin sizes. If violins could be passed along as hand-me-downs, and know-ledge transmitted through demonstration and sharing, what was once paid for could be several times used. It was the economy of multiple learning and sharing. Only one piano was needed, the learner violins were cheap, and passing along technique, repertoire, extras like rosin, strings, cases and bows, all helped keep the cost down.

But, suddenly, I threw a spanner into the works, and the machinery of family instrument-learning came to a surprised halt. My parents now had to find a cello, a cello teacher, and the time, space and money to accom-modate them.

I didn't understand all these considerations at the time and I didn't care. I wanted to play the cello and I was not going to give up. Dad had played up to Grade 6 at school age, and joined the local, and free, youth orchestra in London with his very cheap cello. His beloved instru-ment was piano, though, and it was the piano that took him past Grade 8 and with which he especially identified. He had been a really good pianist, with a love particu-larly for Chopin and Debussy, but had turned down the possibility of music school at eleven because he thought it would stop him playing football. The link from playing piano well to actually becoming a pianist was not an easy or obvious one for him, so he went on to study physics at university. My mother learnt piano past Grade 7 at school but didn't actually take the Grade 8 exam, a fact that became a family joke between my parents. She had been handed a clarinet and free clarinet lessons at school, with which she played in the primary school band and secondary school orchestra. Yet she had always sat and listened to the violin section with transfixed envy, convinced that here, just beyond her reach, was a special and extraordinary knowledge. My unbending determination to play the cello was a shift and a surprise for both parents, but they felt they had no choice but to respond.

The local music shop, Windblowers, recommended a young, gifted, performing cellist who had graduated from the Royal College of Music, Sarah Huson, who told Mum and Dad where to go to get my first cello, a quarter-size rental. Buying smaller cellos wasn't cost-effective because their relative rarity and limited use (I would grow out of it) made them an expensive item. It was more affordable to rent until I grew big enough for a half-size, then three-quarter size, then seven-eighth and finally full-size. But these faraway futures weren't in my head then. I will never forget the excitement of that day, the day I took possession of my very first cello. I stood with it in the 'piano room' at home, not much bigger than the cello was, and touched its cool, wooden front and curled scroll. When I pulled the strings, the sound went through me and filled me in a way the violin never could. From the beginning I felt soothed and befriended by it, not once challenged or in any way scolded by its voice. The cello felt like me.

Music education can begin anywhere, on any instrument. My mother's and sister's first instruments were recorders, and we were all given two main instruments to learn. Deciding what should be 'your' instrument can be entirely accidental, or can feel – as it did in my case – utterly necessary. But music can be learnt in many ways and through many voices. I revelled in the connections and the differences between piano and cello, and the harmony of voices and orchestra. I later learnt to love the trombone for the depth of its sound, and the guitar for its song-like chords. I learnt bass guitar at secondary school, relating it to the grounding, humming cello resonance in an orchestra, and adored piano trio chamber music – piano, violin and cello playing together – the violin moving easily and in its right place in Braimah's hands, while Isata's communion with the piano seemed utterly natural.

I could, perhaps, have played a variety of instruments as my main choice, and what pulled me to the cello may have been a mixture of several things; self-assertion in a family, availability of one-to-one teaching, the excellence of the teacher, and being able to play as a trio with my brother and sister. It all fitted into place. However, there was something that fixed me to that cello stool at the age of six for long periods of time, simply playing, experimenting and practising. Something that required me to sit and put my restless energy only into learning how to make the cello sing in my voice. I can't explain how or why, but the cello chose me.

I was very happy at school. I was surrounded, not only by siblings, but by boys and girls like me who lived in the city, spoke like I did and followed the same rules I followed at home. An accepted mutual respect was implicit and also a widespread admiration for the achievements of others. In my first year at Trinity School, pupils from the years above would perform to the lower years, and we watched dance competitions, singing and several different bands. Most were teacher-led and some put together by pupils. Every lunchtime and often after school, we rehearsed together in orchestras or in various bands for concerts to perform in front of parents, peers, the primary school next door, or the old people's home down the road. There was a piano competition that parents came to, and a big musical, pulling together the skills of aspiring actors, dancers, singers, musicians, set designers, artists, and those adept at textiles and lighting – or simply pupils who wanted to have a go at these things while still in school. Three or four performances were staged over the week, with everyone not involved in the show coming to watch, and the excitement was palpable. The show belonged to all of us.

The effect of collaborations like this, and the extraordinary improvements and outcomes we saw in the performances of other children was life-changing. We all saw our friends, ordinary and just like us, transform themselves into something extraordinary. Those who were, or were not, particularly academic, or sporty, became lauded for their performances onstage, or their achievements as team members. If you *were* very academic, or sporty, it was an extra and even more important achievement to play an instrument, or sing, or act, or dance. The courage needed and the support offered to do these things in school created an atmosphere of mutual pride and appreciation. We all knew each other, somehow. There was a school bond we entered and claimed. And success was never alone.

Nowadays, this kind of music provision is common in private schools, but is extremely rare in the state sector. In December 2016, after I had won BBC Young Musician in the May of that year, our school Prize-giving took place. The school rented Nottingham's Albert Hall, and the concert hall in which I had set my heart on the cello became the place where the whole school gathered to witness the presentation of my award from the headteacher, Mr Dexter, who had replaced Mr McKeever, both incredible and inspirational headteachers who cared passionately about music, and also about each and every pupil, and every pupil's potential, no matter what their particular gifts might be. Both headteachers had been part of the growth of the school into a creative arts school of excellence and both understood how and why the school was so successful. Mike McKeever was ebullient, blunt and always encouraging, full of the belief that everyone could do anything. John Dexter was gentle but authoritative, and would always take the time to stop, look you in the eye and ask how you were. Pupils returned every year in droves for Prize-giving, taking time out of university terms, or training schemes, or jobs for the honour of receiving their exam certificates or prizes from school. It was a time of reunion, appreciation, and usually a good night out in Nottingham after the ceremony. We were even lucky enough to host Julian Lloyd Webber as guest speaker. Julian had been one of the judges in the BBC Young Musician String Category Final, and had been in touch with me ever since, offering his support and interest. To have the friendship and advice of such a famous and well-respected cellist was incredible for someone like me who had, less than a year ago, been playing in small concerts at school and at the Junior Academy, watching and admiring 'real' cellists like Julian Lloyd Webber from afar. Mike McKeever, before stepping down as headteacher, had simply decided to make a request for Julian to speak at the Prize-giving, and to everyone's astonishment, he said yes. Julian handed out prizes and A-level certificates, giving an uplifting address to everyone there, making us even prouder of the school we belonged to. I still remember his generous speech and his praise of Trinity as the ideal blueprint for a successful school, committed to music. He had to remind himself that this was an ordinary, diverse, city comprehensive, and not a prestigious fee-paying school, and as he wrote in *The Strad*: 'What hope do we have of shedding the "elitist" tag if only those with rich parents get to learn an instrument at school?'[6] The pupils here were lucky. And the evident dividing line this exposes in education and opportunity still makes me sad.

Music education cannot be left to rest on the random distribution of luck. I never take my luck for granted, but I also don't want it ring-fenced for a minority who happen to be in the right place at the right time, with the right family and the right school. I'm referring to the luck not only of becoming a cellist, or a professional musician, but of having access to music as a schoolchild, which is an access that reverberates through a lifetime.

Access, and by extension choice, involves the removal of cultural stigmas and entrenched ideas and preconceptions of music as a subject. Music is both theoretical and practical – like science or applied mathematics. It does require application, commitment and practice, as well as historical enquiry, linguistic skills and geographical understanding. Without a goal of progress, competence and rigorous learning, however, any subject can become 'dumbed-down' and lacking in focus or structure. If it is only children from one social class, or one ethnic background, or one type of school, who have the privilege of enjoying a high standard of music education and instrumental lessons, then music becomes, by default, elitist.

What I saw at school were children from all backgrounds whose natural talent for music was stoked into a desire to learn, perform and improve, who found joy and confidence from the camaraderie of playing or singing in unison, and learning new kinds of music together. Being good at music was praised, and it was possible, even probable that, like me, you could be in the football team and in the boys' choir, and play a musical instrument, without having to choose one identity over another. Joining in, getting better and gaining a voice led only to an increase in self-esteem and friendship across the school community.

The grand piano in the Lower School Hall had been donated to the school, apparently by a member of the Steinway family. In her first year, Isata won two digital pianos for the school in the Clement Pianos Nottinghamshire Pianist competition. The competition was actually changed after this initial year, no longer offering the school piano prize because most school music departments in the area simply didn't tell their pupils about it, claiming they had no one in the school advanced enough to compete. For Trinity to put forward the winning pupil in a competition almost exclusively dominated by the private schools, was testament to its sense of undoubted mutual belief and communal expectation.

One of my favourite groups, very popular with those of us in the football team, was the steel pans, and we always performed at school concerts. The only expectations here were enthusiasm and natural musicality.

Developing a strong sense of rhythm alongside melody and harmony is a requisite and an effect of playing steel pans. I thought of the rocking, bouncing lorries in Antigua on J'ouvert Morning, and the road vibrating through my shoes with the rising sun before I could even see them. This was what I wanted to do. To get under the skin and through the very soles of people's feet before they were aware of what was happening. Standing shoulder to shoulder with friends I saw daily, I would try to match my rhythm to theirs, and to blend my pitch in irresistible harmony between their sounds. So intense was the concentration needed for this that we were listening to each other on a knife-edge, borne along on a tide of rules we could neither break nor refuse. I alternated between the pans, the bass guitar, cello and voice, and entered the piano competition for my house team at the start of every year.

I didn't know how unusual this kind of schooling was for children like us. I probably didn't even think about it. I just assumed that all state schools achieved this integration between pupils and staff, and across ethnicities. I thought all schools enjoyed this unified vision of shared success and ambition, with music as its expression. The fragility of this system, regardless of its measurable outcomes, was a shock to me. Wasn't it obvious, evidential even, that it worked?

I won BBC Young Musician at the age of seventeen, in Year 12. By the time that I was nearly eighteen and in

Year 13, Mr Dexter, our brilliant headteacher, left and was replaced by another. With him came a very new school structure and leadership. Trinity no longer had budgetary independence but had been subsumed under a Multi-Academy Trust. This forced the different Catholic schools of varying visions and success in Nottinghamshire under one umbrella and with one 'super-Head'. The individual school headteachers now lost any overarching financial and cultural governance, and the schools were forced into a one-size-fits-all package.

However, one size did not fit all. Trinity's ethos became subject to a greater power.

I remember the visceral shock when we witnessed a host of music teachers losing their jobs. The cello teacher left and was deliberately not replaced, even though a new group of young players had begun to have lessons, inspired to see what was possible in their own environment. The school show was cancelled and Prize-giving – the school's biggest musical collaboration – banned until, eventually, a shrunken version was allowed to happen in the sports hall. School concerts were difficult to put on because of the time they took to organize, and the number of music and other subject teachers who needed to be involved. There were fewer visiting music teachers and the price of instrument lessons went up. The school said that music was still a priority, but these effects of the funding cuts gave the impression that music got in the way of the 'real' business of school.

There was resistance. The head of drama, Mrs White, having been forbidden to put on the annual school show due to copyright costs, wrote her own script and cor-ralled support from the remaining music and dance departments to stage a show, regardless. The staff and pupils felt defiant. The usual large number of children and teenagers across school years took part and learnt a script full of references to the unbending force of the creative arts, and enacted a plot dedicated to the triumph of self-expression over silence. But the dance studio, a room apart and kept free for learning and practising dance choreography and dance lessons, was discon-tinued and ripped open to became part of the dining area for an ever-increasing school population. The school instrument stock, built up and looked after over time, lost its maintenance budget. Violins and cellos became stringless, bows lacked hair, the drum section developed patches and holes, brass and woodwind instruments lost valves and reeds. In the following years, the decreasing budget for state schools led to a catastrophic leak in the roof above the music room, resulting in the irreversible loss of many musical instruments, not replaced by the new school governance.

Just after winning BBC Young Musician at seventeen, I had joined the school trip to Lourdes as my penulti-mate year was nearing its end. In Lourdes, the idea of giving, loving and communicating was embedded in our venture to help others in a pilgrimage to face and relieve suffering, and our nights were full of music-making. A new world was opening up to me, made possible by a school which had wrapped itself around me and cheered me on. In the autumn of the next year, I would be a student at the Royal Academy of Music, studying cello with Hannah Roberts, a dream that should have been impossible from where I came, and might become impossible for those that tried to follow.

I was sad to see the deepening gloom of a school becoming increasingly powerless to nurture its own pupils. I couldn't bear the stories I heard, first-hand from my younger sisters, of friends who had taken up the cello following my BBC Young Musician win, just coming into the initial school orchestra and ensembles, and finding their cello teacher gone with no replacement. They were bewildered, not sure where to put their new-found excitement and enthusiasm, and unable to afford private lessons or a cello outside school. They were simply dropping out of music altogether. There was one moment of defiance and compassion I could still manage, clear that this was a gesture, a demonstration and a statement as much as I hoped it would be a small bridge of support for those pupils I wanted to bring with me. My prize for winning BBC Young Musician was three thousand pounds and all I had to give. So I donated it to Trinity to fund a cello teacher for three more years. I had just signed with Decca Classics, who offered to match-fund this gift and give the same amount. It was a thank you, a recognition of what

I had been given, and a farewell gesture like a bouquet of flowers against a coming storm. The great question was, how can one individual effect change?

Proof of the role of music education in forming and informing young minds, its powerful role in developing intelligence, communication skills, discipline and mutual respect in children and schools, is well documented. I can also outline my own direct experiences, those of other musicians, and people who have benefited from learning music, yet education policy continues to pull out music by the roots.

Eminent musicians are repeatedly giving first-hand evidence of the importance of music for young people and for people throughout life, and painstakingly outlining the threads that tie music education with individual as well as societal outcomes. Jess Gillam, the renowned saxophonist, has put forward numerous statements in support of music education. In a letter to the *Guardian* she claimed that 'learning an instrument can teach so many fundamental life skills. It promotes discipline, empathy, determination and cooperation as well as providing a sense of community and worth.'[7] And yet, the current situation is hurtling fast in the opposite direction: 'We are reaching a crisis point. We are in danger of crushing creativity, innovation and expression.'

If we need guidance on the science behind music education, there are countless research documents and analyses behind this. For example, findings by Samata

Sharma and David Silbersweig demonstrate that 'musical training over time has been shown to increase the connectivity of certain brain regions'.[8,9] The paper's abstract reveals the scope of the research: 'The very fact that music is processed by so many areas of the brain (ranging from the cortex, to the limbic system, to the neuroendocrine and even autonomic nervous systems), exerts an effect not only on our brain, but also on our bodies . . . and can thereby shape our individual brain structure and function to mitigate collective disease severity and improve wellness across populations.'[10,11]

But scientific research, medicine, and the assertions of respected musicians, as well as evidence on the ground, are regularly pushed outside the boundaries of education policy. Published in 2022, the National Plan for Music Education, 'The Power of Music to Change Lives', is a worthy and welcome statement of intent for music education in England. The Plan recognizes that 'music is an essential part of a broad and ambitious curriculum for all pupils. It must not be the preserve of the privileged few'.[12] Curriculum music, mandatory at one hour a week, is important, as well as the emphasis on inclusion, a broad range of music – including a solid and diverse introduction to classical music, and an acknowledgement that music education serves a range of purposes from well-being, developing creativity, and the foundation of a career in music. The references to inclusion come with the list of classical composers to be studied, including long-forgotten or sidelined Black and women composers, for example, Samuel Coleridge-Taylor, Anna Clyne and Anna Meredith, music from around the world, the statement that children with special educational needs need specialist support, and the understanding that progression in music will need to be backed up by funding for disadvantaged children.

I read the Plan with real optimism, but when I turn to the reality of music education in schools I despair. Firstly, is one hour a week really impactful, or even noticeable? Secondly, both the Musicians' Union and the Independent Society of Musicians point to the strangely elliptical nature of funding in music education. The Plan is delivered by Music Hubs of varying success around England to which schools apply for partnership. Many schools do not engage with their Hub at all and there appears to be little or no enforcement to do this. Even if they do apply for partnership with the Hubs, the inadequate financial backing makes music education a questionable pursuit for many schools.

My own experience of music education makes me nonplussed and confused by the system now, but I can witness the results, both anecdotally and through my younger sisters' experiences, and they seem to be uneven and frighteningly patchy. In an open letter to the then Education Secretary, Gillian Keegan, in December 2023, several music education organizations pointed to the financial gap between stated intention and delivery:

'On current funding levels [. . .] many organizations within Hubs are finding themselves struggling to identify which areas of activity to cut next.'[13] The conclusion fits with what I frequently witness in many of the state schools I visit: 'In its National Plan for Music Education, the Government has asked the music education sector to deliver more than ever, and yet it has offered no increase in funding for well over a decade.'

There appears to be a trench dug between the stated duties of the Hubs to deliver the Plan for music education, and enforcement – or incentive – for the schools themselves to accept it. Conflicting accountability for schools to implement core subjects, STEM, the English Baccalaureate and Progress 8 measures, all pit schools fundamentally against music, and anyway, the Plan is 'non-statutory guidance'.[14] A school would need to have gritty determination to hold up and use its scanty budget for music in the face of government accountability, and parental pressure, for delivering a good standard of education. I loved maths at school, and was passionate about the subject, but valued my right to love music too and not to have to pitch one against the other in a bitter struggle of 'either-or'.

Richard Morrison makes the vital observation about the National Plan for Music Education: 'If all the inequalities and patchiness of music education in England could be solved by fine words, this document would be perfect.'[15] But, fundamentally, before we talk about resources, or scientific enquiry, or musical expertise, or lived experience, we need to identify the philosophy and ideals behind current education policy in a world aggressively devoted to business, profit and computation. As Richard Morrison points out: 'I have rarely met a music teacher, professional musician or musically aware parent who can't identify the problems. They boil down to one thing: disrespect. Music is still belittled as an academic subject. Consequently it is starved of curriculum time, trained teachers and resources.'

Music education cannot be delivered without its practitioners and without training music teachers. With music starved from the curriculum and, more significantly, with the value of music disastrously undermined, where will the workforce – properly esteemed, nurtured and skilled – come from? Dr Ally Daubney identifies this key issue: 'The trouble is, we just don't have enough music teachers, there are increasingly casualized workforce models that do not support the development of music teachers and we are already in a time of crisis as far as music teacher recruitment, training and retention is concerned.'[16]

And, to ask the central question, I leave it to Richard Morrison: 'What about the small matter of money?'

I am Patron of Music Masters and Ambassador for Future Talent, and I've worked with these charities and others since my teens. These organizations shouldn't have to exist at all and they are evidence of the widening gap between need and provision in music services. Music Masters works with a number of UK schools with a large intake of disadvantaged pupils, and staff keen to offer a high level of music teaching. The emphasis is on instrument-learning, on staff training and support, and on providing a continuous path of advancement on a child's instrument of choice. Importantly, Music Masters lights the fire of children's interest and delight in learning to play, and stays with them through school and beyond, even offering postgraduate degrees in music teaching and continued mentoring after graduation. In their own words: 'Music as a core subject is being lost. Music Masters work at a school level because it is the clearest way to reach children of all backgrounds, where we model what a high-quality music education can look like in every school.'

Future Talent raises funds to help children access instrument-learning outside school, to take up places, for example, at Saturday conservatoires and to be loaned good instruments to play. Their target group is the 'gifted young musicians' who need the extra financial and teaching support not otherwise open to them: 'We break down barriers, create opportunities and harness the power of music to transform the lives of young musicians across the UK.'

I am glad to be involved in both initiatives as they address different areas of my own music education and reveal what it takes not only to have access to music, but to become a musician. And it begins early.

It's quickly obvious to all parents or guardians who try to give children a good music education that learning a musical instrument outside school is an expensive undertaking. The mounting costs faced by my parents came from not only the cost of lessons but also the price of instrument purchase or hire, which got steeper the older we became and the bigger or better instruments we needed. Maintaining instruments was another ongoing cost. Focusing on the instruments we played, pianos need tuning, and violins, violas and cellos need replacement strings, and rosin to warm and release the sound of the bow. The bows, whose quality matters the more advanced you get, and which becomes increasingly expensive to achieve, also needs regular re-hairing. Instruments need repairs: bridges need to be replaced, cracks glued, sound-posts repositioned, and the skilled luthiers who do this work need to be paid. Then there's the cost of travelling to lessons, or courses, or concerts, and the music scores that have to be bought. The price of entering competitions and festivals to develop performance craft and the clothes and shoes needed for those performances are all part of the balance-sheet, and that's before we factor in concert tickets to watch live music. My parents often talk about the cost of funding concert tickets for the family to watch each other at our own performances, a price that seemed to spiral year on year!

But, of course, it's not just money that's an issue – although that can be the biggest barrier of all. It's also expertise and time. It's having access to knowledge. How do we do this? Who is going to give us advice? What is this all about, really? Guidance, inspiration and recommendations count for a lot.

The first time I entered a school not as a pupil but as someone invited to inspire other pupils, I was thirteen. I arrived at Gallions Primary in East London, not much taller than my cello. I had been asked by Roz Deville, then music manager at the school (now CEO of Music Masters), to play to these young primary school children. They had been given the great gift of a host of stringed instruments – cellos and violins – and some group teaching to learn to play. I was so impressed that children in a school like this could have the chance to play cellos all together with their friends that it took my breath away.

I walked into the school hall and, in a hushed circle, sat about ten little cellists, many of them from African-Caribbean or South Asian backgrounds. Several faces with big, watchful eyes waited, looking expectantly at me, their quarter-size cellos held in front of them, vibrant with excitement. My knees felt strangely weak with the sudden sense of huge responsibility. I had the job of taking all this expectation which was shining before me, and somehow revealing the wonder they watched for.

This task was nothing less than drawing back a curtain and showing the possibilities before them on a journey they had barely started. Through instruction, demonstration and patience, these cellos had to sing for them.

And they did. Amazingly, note by note, with a thrill that never dropped, we drew our bows together over single strings. We were a chorus, moving step-by-step in a unison possible through music. I knew this was a communion enacted in the special concentration that comes of teasing sound and meaning from an instrument. They were learning to play. And I was full of delight.

When I performed for them all, they sat cross-legged on the floorboards and listened with their entire bodies, not missing a note, a string, a move of wrist or finger. I played and watched them in simultaneous fascination, honoured by their unflinching attention, and brimming with the energy they gave me. I never forgot the sheer, abandoned joy on the faces of those primary school children and the applause that I received. And many of those children have continued to learn and play, and to perform in their turn.

I have spent time with many classes of children and young people since then, and it's the most rewarding work I do, and still amongst the most demanding. Because of this, and because of the teaching I have been so lucky to receive, I retain unbounded respect for music teachers. Music teaching is a position of great responsibility and trust. It requires energy, dedication and concentration.

Particularly, it demands an intense watchfulness to the personality and needs of the person in front of you. There is no 'one-size-fits-all' when it comes to teaching, even if you have the short, bounded time of a master-class or group lesson.

With a young person next to or facing me, I always have a powerful sense of privilege. I have been allowed into that intensely personal space where someone is grappling with the interpretation of a piece of music and, at the same time, wrestling with the demands of their own voice. Learning to balance the requirements and nuances of a composer's intention with the urgent individuality of your own expression – your own joy, pain, delight – is a process steeped in vulnerability as well as curiosity.

I take my role as guide and advisor very seriously. Effective teaching calls for an intense awareness of the significance of what you say to a young person at a specific stage of exploration and development. It calls for an unnerving balance between encouragement and firmness, licence and clarity. In a masterclass, my role is to enter for a brief moment someone else's trek on the long road of learning an instrument and finding one's own place in music and performance, and I have to be realistic about what I can achieve in that time. What will be enough to cause that thrill of achievement and feeling of progress here and now? What will be enough to spark the next few steps of learning, or to steady the direction to the next goal?

Many masterclasses are in front of an audience, and here lies another element of responsibility. The young person I am teaching is also performing, revealing their strengths and weaknesses, their ability to listen, improve, impress, be worth the attention. I am given the task to listen in depth, to calm nerves and egos, and to decide in a moment what is either most needed from me musically and technically, or what is most valuable to praise, enhance and coax. It's about the person in the moment, and about the music. But, crucially, it's not about me.

In 2022 I became Menuhin Visiting Professor of Performance Mentoring at the Royal Academy of Music. In this position, I meet young musicians at different stages in their relationship with music. As undergraduates or postgraduates, they have made the decision to dedicate a major part – perhaps all – of their lives to playing the cello. Their goals are both personal and professional. They may be hoping for careers in an orchestra, chamber group, teaching, artist or arts management, or as soloists. But my task is to listen to their engagement with a piece of music, to understand their personality in the music and the performance and to enter a conversation with them, often from my cello to theirs. It's a space of great privilege, seriousness and hope.

4. Equality or Quality?

My childhood with six siblings was full of games, out-
doors and indoors. We climbed trees, played football
and chased each other up hills and through forests.
We challenged each other to board games, schemed
imaginatively behind our parents' backs, and built intricate castles together out of scrap paper and cardboard.
Mealtimes were loud and crowded, bedtimes busy and
communication always competing and always noisy.

We were let loose to play with free, creative abandon
and our personalities bounced off and deeply influenced
each other in a raucous intimacy we all shared. Our
play was infused with energy but structured by rules. It
mattered that we played our games with commitment.
Whatever artwork we made, or dance routine we formed
together, or race we took part in, had to be done with all
our concentration and all our might.

And that's how we approached our music.

I didn't just want to play the cello to join in and have
fun. I wanted to play well. I wanted to learn every technique I could to produce the sounds and feelings I didn't
yet even know I had. I had an insatiable curiosity, and I
wanted to play excellently.

I couldn't rest until I had worked out how to make a long note flow as the same note even through a change of bow direction. I would sit for whole evenings, although they seemed timeless, until my fingers moved fast enough to master a passage of fast quavers. And that pure vibrato voice, climbing higher and higher in crescendo, to its heart-rending top note in the first movement of Elgar's cello concerto, which had to be unforgettable.

If there hadn't been space for that curiosity to drive me at its own, blazing speed, I would have become frustrated, restless, perhaps even bored. Learning the cello in a lukewarm, uncommitted way would have been meaningless, and to be held back, humiliating.

Sitting in the waiting room before my Grade 3 cello exam at the age of seven, I was so impatient to play, I started my imitation of Jacqueline du Pré playing the Elgar concerto and remained in full performance before it was time to go in. The possible – and to me, inevitable – future was in my head already and I inhabited each note with the bravado of the famous cellist fronting a full orchestra. I imagined that my half-size cello was du Pré's fabulous Davidov Stradivarius, and that I could play anything.

The important thing was, no one told me I couldn't. No one laughed or looked incredulous when I said I would be a cellist. My parents and teachers didn't tell me to wake up and realize it was an impossible dream or that I was incapable. And they were always willing to facilitate my desire to learn.

Music education in childhood and in school should be a cornerstone of every child's life and a universal right. We talk of universal literacy, or the general right to education of every person, whether refugee or citizen, from whatever background, religion or means. And therefore, the issue of what constitutes education and whether that constitution should be equally distributed remains critical.

But if we're going to talk about music and education, we also have to talk about excellence. We need to talk about what we mean by progress, by talent, by drive, and by ambition. How do we discuss equality and *also* excellence? What about those children and young people who don't just want to join in and have a go, but want to be advanced on their instruments? What about those children and teenagers who want to go on to higher education with music, and/or want to be professional musicians? How about those who may one day want to choose to work in the music industry in a capacity they may not yet know exists? What does equal opportunity mean if we put it next to aspiration and success?

I think it's important to talk about encouraging and nurturing children in music but we have to find a balance between encouragement and judgement. At some point in every subject and in every sport, those who want to learn and train seriously need to be given the chance to work seriously, and to face appraisal. When do we cross the fine line between positive reinforcement and negative enforcement? These are particularly tricky questions in music, because it's possible to make music at so many different levels, and for so many different reasons. Are we emphasizing fun or work? Is music a free-for-all leisure activity with no reference to achievement, or an exercise in discipline?

Charities, teachers, parents and schools can face difficulty and even embarrassment when they attempt to confront these issues. For example, if there is a chance to learn an instrument as part of the school curriculum, should teachers provide any platform for competition or pathways for examinations? Should charities offer intensive lessons for those who want to improve quickly, and can parents insist that their children take on a dedicated or routine practice regime?

I have discussed the unifying force of music and how music in schools fosters community, self-esteem and teamwork. I recognize the importance of nurturing musicality in everyone and giving everyone access to equally distributed instruction and collaboration in music. But in all areas of education we rely on selection and ranking. We include testing, exams, competition and selection to reward advancement or to recognize exception. Striving to succeed or to exceed is part of society, culture and schooling. What is its place in music?

As a child, my education in music was not primarily or exclusively within my state school. My parents were passionate about music and determined to give all their seven children a chance to obtain the highest standards we could on our instruments. For them, being parents of Black children meant a keen understanding that nothing could be taken for granted. My mother said – after I became an adult – that complacency had never been an option. They both knew that opportunities were not going to fall into our laps without effort and hard work. There were no guarantees of doors opening and rolling happily into the certainty of a successful career. This was a difficult reality, and often frustrating, but in the management of my parents, it became empowering. Achievement demanded endeavour and to be kind of OK on our instruments was to be entirely invisible.

The first, and most obvious, barrier was money. Outside state education, music and instrument-learning is often prohibitively expensive, so to set out on this path, you have to really mean it. A tepid approach would be a waste of money. So why was it necessary at all? My parents recognized that music and instrument-learning couldn't wait until a school curriculum or individual school deemed it time to offer a group lesson or provide an instrument it had in stock. They did ask about violin lessons in my primary school but these couldn't begin until Year 5, when pupils are aged nine and ten, and we were all alert and ready to learn years before that. My parents were also aware that time and age are crucial in the world of music. To have the chance to become a virtuoso, or even to have a job as a working classical musician, starting to learn piano or a stringed instrument from scratch at nine or ten years old risks beginning too late.

My parents had two very useful resources at their disposal. One was knowledge and training enough to start us on piano and violin and teach us to a certain level before paying for instrument teachers. The other was the courage to sacrifice other essential acquirements (house and car maintenance, heating and home decoration) and buy a piano. And that, after all, is the engine of education. The ideals and the philosophy – what is prized and valued – drive the priorities and goals that are fought for.

Our parents wanted us not only to have the opportunity to *learn* music, but the opportunity to *excel* in music. These are not necessarily the same things. In fact, these are often not at all the same things. If you put limits and boundaries around what a talented child can explore in music, and how far they can go, it can be a deprivation as harsh as complete denial. We have to assume, without prejudging, that every child has talent and can develop the desire to excel. And that assumption involves expectation. If we expect certain children and not others to achieve excellence in music, we simultaneously denounce and destroy the chances of those we decide are incapable.

This is where policy-makers in the state sector become uncomfortable. People worry that, surely, expectation is the twin curse of parental or societal pressure. Instead of encouragement, doesn't expecting a child to be able to succeed risk the shame of failure? It seems that schools have accepted music's links with well-being and are able to teach it in a way that emphasizes freedom and exploration, but at the cost of encouraging serious hard work. Diligent practice in music is often associated with anxiety and misery. Some educators seem to consider the expectation to excel as something of a prison sentence. But the irony is that, if I had not been expected to excel, and had not been given the tools to know how to practise and become advanced on the cello, my potential would have dripped away – and that, to me, would have felt like prison.

I have spoken publicly about the difference between expectation and pressure. While I was being interviewed on BBC Radio 4 for *Desert Island Discs*, Lauren Laverne asked me whether parental expectation was a lot for a child to cope with, and a heavy burden to bear.[1] This was an interesting perspective for me to consider because for me and my siblings, our parents' expectations of us were a great gift in a world that, in general, expected little of us. To be quietly accepted as not only capable but also certain of achievement was a rebuttal against a myriad negative reinforcements outside our home. Expectation was a charm we were given to clutch and a talisman against defeat.

My answer was to draw a distinction between on the one hand, a kind of loving recognition and on the other, the misery of relentless and unrealistic demands. An exhortation to reach one's potential is an olive branch in a world where what you can't or shouldn't do is in restless flood beneath you. And expectation means responsibility on both sides. If my parents had expected little of us, their task as parents would have been remarkably simple. There would have been little point in exerting energy to a job that seemed impossible, or wasting time and money on someone not likely to achieve much more than a fleeting moment of pleasure in an occupation inevitably out of reach. And for me and my siblings, it would have been very hard to know how to open a door marked 'Impossible', and enter through it.

Our parents considered us worthy of financial sacrifice and monumental parental effort. And our school teachers were willing to reinforce this. My sister Isata always talks about her primary school class teacher, Grace Cracknell, who would ask her to play the piano in assembly. When Isata told her at the age of eight that she wanted to be a concert pianist, she neither flinched nor missed a beat but simply said, 'Yes, work hard and you will be.' For Isata, that second of time was a shining moment she still carries with her. And what if she had instead been dismissed, and given derision instead of acceptance? Or an amused raising of the eyebrows? I think of all those children in similar circumstances turned away, not with the warmth of calm optimism but, while in the centre of all that bright possibility, a cold bullet of disbelief.

I often worry about this confusion of meritocracy with mediocrity. A truly equal music education allows everyone to compete at the highest level for the outcome they dream and hope for. And that is not the same as saying that everyone will achieve that highest goal, or that everyone wants to be a musician, ultimately. We were always told, with candour, that excellence is within everyone's reach if given the chance, but that it has a price, and that price is hard work. And if everyone is to have an equal chance to excel, we all deserve that honesty.

Not many children naturally choose hard work over fun, and there's great skill in demonstrating that one leads to the other. When we were given lessons at home from Mum or Dad, it wasn't always fun, or at least, it wasn't always a welcome summons. I liked kicking my football, painting pictures, building structures out of cardboard and glue, or practising somersaults on the hallway rug. The garden outside smelt of grass and mud, and emitted the tantalizing aroma of cricket with a plastic ball. I enjoyed illicitly clambering on the garage roof with my brother, Braimah, or catapulting down the stairs on cushions pulled from the settee. Listening to rap music on the stereo or playing hide-and-seek in the dark with my brother and sisters: these things were all easy fun. The parental call to the piano stool was an unwelcome interruption and I became adept at 'not hearing' the call when it was my turn. Although I loved to play the piano, I've never relished the abrupt disruption of a glorious game.

But I would nevertheless be plucked from whatever joyous adventure I was steeped in and placed, unceremoniously, on that stool, a stool of which I have very clear memories. It's since become irretrievably broken but has never been thrown away. It's kept somewhere amongst the bric-a-brac in the garage, too sentimentally precious for my mum to lose. Apparently, my Welsh great-grandfather either made it from scratch or reconstituted it from another broken piano stool. It may have been the same stool my grandmother was made to sit on when she was practising piano chords in a cold front room in Cardiff or Newport. Her father had sawn a piece of wood for the seat and covered it in a piece of old leather ripped from perhaps a car seat, or an old settee. He had attached leather straps to make the seat into a lid that could be propped up, under which my mum's old recorder and clarinet books were mysteriously stored. The height wasn't adjustable so as a small child, my parents found a cushion for me to sit on, making me high enough to reach the keys comfortably. And there, from the age of five, I would find myself, expected to steady my mind and concentrate on the keyboard in front of me, allowing my thoughts to follow the tactile sounds my fingers made. Once there, concentrating and concentrated on, I shone as the centre of something special, in the peace of learning and exploration, held in communion with my own endless possibilities.

We are in danger of patronizing children from certain backgrounds when we take steps to protect them from the rigours of hard work, the strictures of disciplined practice, or the risks of exposure. Perhaps it depends on the words we use. I've spoken already about how classical music is often associated with a kind of terror in the popular imagination. There is the terror of perfection, where, many people think, classical musicians must strive for the holy grail of flawless playing. The word 'competition' is often aligned with the terror of comparison with others, and performance often viewed as the spotlight of judgement. Exams bring to mind censure and criticism, being tested and found wanting. And right here lurks the fear of failure.

We need to explore and re-evaluate the idea of failure. If we don't allow children to test themselves, we teach them to fear – and to even expect – failure. And yet failure is a reality all children need to learn to face, to assess and to deal with. The terror of failure can't be avoided without experiencing it more than once. Mistakes, losing, not being 'the best', and not being 'good enough' are all stones on the road to success.

My own experience of music exams was positive because they were an external method of measuring my achievement and telling me how far and fast I was advancing. They were like steps on a ladder and pin-nacles to keep in my mind's eye. I took Grades 1 to 8 on piano and cello, missing out the odd grade here and there but making sure I kept the order of con-stant progression. Each grade tested me by presenting more difficult and advanced pieces to learn, three pieces for each exam, to be played live in the presence of an examiner. Each piece tested a different style of playing, roughly arranged by era and historical time. Put simply, I would have to play a baroque piece, from the eighteenth century; one from the nineteenth-century Romantic era; and a twentieth-century piece. In addition, I had to play scales and arpeggios when the keys were called out; I'd be tested aurally, on my ability to discuss music and chords by ear only; and have sight-reading tests, in which I had to play a piece from a score I'd never seen before. Grade exams were a comprehensive test of my musical ability and command of the instrument, as well as my ability to perform live. On the cello, a piano accompan-ist, often either my cello teacher or Isata, would join me and the test included how well I played in ensemble with them.

These steps on a ladder were proof that I was getting better – but this doesn't mean I didn't stumble and fall from time to time. Learning to deal with the nerves like a lightning rod through the body when it's your turn to walk into the exam room and perform in front of the examiner was part of the deal. The physical discomfort of arrival at that eleventh hour when finally there would be nowhere to hide was a fact. That scale that should have been practised to fluency would be forced, limping into the light of day. And the responsibility was entirely your own. At the age of seven, for example, having not bothered myself unduly with preparation, paying little attention to the practice papers I should have completed, and feeling happily free from apprehension, I sauntered into my written Grade 4 music theory exam, and failed.

Performance was a state of being that I enjoyed. Being watched as I showed what I had to express through the piano or cello felt like a privilege and a release. However, this privilege came with responsibility. There is no joy in finding yourself onstage and completely unprepared for the task. Learning the meaning of adequate preparation is a lesson in time management, projection and planning. And then the moment of performance unfolds as a long-awaited delight rather than a plunging panic. Inevitably – and probably, admittedly usefully – I learnt this the hard way.

Formal speech caused me more problems and came less naturally to me. I found aural tests as simple as mental maths, with everything mapped out before me in obvious patterns. But in my Grade 8 cello exam, I blurted out the wrong answer, realized immediately what I had done but didn't know how to form the words to correct the response. At the age of nine, it seemed unsurmountable to express in words any extra sentence, so I let my silence swallow me up and felt the examiner's wide-eyed surprise linger as I withdrew.

A form of kindness lives, not in protecting children from jeopardy, but in letting them develop the expertise to face it, in all its guises. And that's why I'm an advocate of music festivals. We were regular participants in local music festivals, which are days, or a clutch of days, or a week, of rolling competitive classes. My parents would enter each of us into a range of classes, based on our grade level, or our age, or genre, or length of piece. We would often take part in chamber or duo classes, compete on both our instruments, and if they didn't clash, we would watch each other's performances.

Music festival classes were not expensive when taken individually, but they must have mounted into real expenditure after multiple age groups, grades and pieces were entered by our growing family. The more advanced we got, the more expensive it was to enter, but my parents knew how valuable these days were, and carried on filling in the endless paper forms and categories. They also never divulged any of the costs to us. We had no idea that anything was required except our preparation and practice. I didn't for one moment think about money or administrative time but only about my turn onstage. So much had to be learnt the hard way.

One year, I insisted on entering several pieces in back-to-back classes, full of the hubris of performance. I could almost taste the thrill of being able to face, in full instrumental voice, that audience of parents, children and the general public, repeating the joy of being in the centre of attention. I could already feel the cool silver and brass of the trophies I would win, but the real prize, the point of bliss, came with the final pull of bow on string, the triumphant fling, arm above head, as the audience applauded.

The issue was that, at the age of ten or eleven, I struggled to keep all those pieces at the apex of my concentration. Performance requires a level of fluency and being able to play the music so well that it's almost second nature. This guards against the unexpected fluctuations of a live, anything-can-happen environment. The random coughing in the audience, the unfamiliar cello stool, the distraction of a slightly out-of-tune piano, an unnervingly skilful competitor playing directly before you: all this has to be managed by the physical and mental trust built up through recurrent and deepening knowledge of the repertoire. Body and mind work like an oiled machine if a piece of music is practised to the right level and focus.

But I had stretched myself too thin. Chasing glory, I tripped up on the details and found myself floundering. Instead of the fluid energy I was used to, leading to the unmitigated triumph of the final flourish, my mind was glitching, coming up short against decisions I wasn't sure how to make and directions that left me confused. I got through it, patching together harmonies and improvising moments that could have been right but weren't quite. I knew I was 'styling it out' rather than enacting the brilliance I sought, and it infuriated me. I realize now that what my parents were revealing afterwards in their lack of words wasn't tight-lipped disappointment, but, flooded with relief that I hadn't been given the trophies I didn't deserve, they knew there was no need for them to speak at all. These were nuances I understood when I was older, of course, and I was able subsequently to fit this into the story of my development as a cellist. As a child, I wanted to win everything and I burnt with disappointment that I couldn't and didn't. But my parents knew that winning is the end goal of a much longer odyssey and winning without deserving to win just leads to the inevitable reckoning at a later date. But on this occasion, I learnt my lesson.

The music festivals and competitions we entered taught us the pitfalls and dangers of preparation – or inadequate preparation – and performance. We all hung over that precipice of memory loss, fighting to find the next note in the wild, white second while the whole world is staring, and failing. We all faced the scramble to recover while semiquavers seemed to fall through the grip of our bow or fingers; and every one of us forgot, at least once, the name of the piece we were about to play at the precise time of announcement. I know, intimately, the sinking hole in the stomach when you realize you have left the piano part for your cello sonata at home on the bed. I feel, still, the blistering sound of the snapping string when there are no spares in the case. And the long, never-ending experience of playing a piano duet with Braimah, when neither of us could catch up with the galloping, nervous speed of our own fingers, and we sweated our way to a disastrous finish. This lives for ever in my memory, alongside the disappointed and sporadic applause that followed.

There is, of course, another side to this. Successfully educating a child hinges on the intermittent or heavily anticipated points of approbation, encouragement and praise that thread through a learning experience allowing children to meet challenges with hope and confidence. Semantics do matter, of course. Or maybe it's tone, body language and attitude that determine the positive effects of setting children up to face the possibility of success. Using words like fear, defeat and failure can be more kindly replaced. Fear is translatable into anticipation, excitement and adrenaline. You can turn defeat into experience and try again. And, knowing that appreciation is the hook for effort, my parents would always try to find something to praise.

Crucially, children need to develop a sense of humour – even if this is rarely associated with classical music and serious musical education. It is perfectly healthy to look back at a performance, an exam or a competition that went less than well and laugh about it. Often distance in time is needed, and often it's a question of looking back from a higher stage of advancement, with things 'going right' scattered in the intervening space. It's a recognition of subsequent triumph, that something important was learnt and that you are taller and stronger because of it. This is the path to generosity and to understanding others, and it's another crucial element in music. Acknowledging the fallible, learning, changing self that requires risk and failure to achieve pinpoint moments of success leads us to empathy. If music education is not about pulling others alongside you on the lurching path to excellence, it leads to extraordinary loneliness.

Music is important precisely because it teaches students to strive for excellence. The idea of testing yourself and putting yourself into a challenging environment where you may be measured against others or judged for your own abilities, preparation and effort, is an idea that must not go out of fashion in the state system. Particularly in the arts and in sport, this emphasis on measurement or goals is being approached with greater nervousness and shied away from in many school environments. Perhaps the move towards making music more of a peripheral subject is stripping it of its claim to serious endeavour. Teamwork and self-esteem are fine attributes but the goal of excellence in any sphere also demands testing, judgement and hard work.

Leaving aside the division between private and state schools, it seems mysterious to me how pride and self-confidence, and that maligned word, ambition, can be nurtured in children without some element of resolve and diligence. For me, there is a great risk in condescending to children in the state sector and thereby denying them the dignity of challenging themselves. I have been astonished, on many occasions, whether as a child, student or professional, at the progress made by someone else in a short space of time. I remember winning a trophy at a music festival, returning the following year, and finding that my competitor of the year before was transformed. They had become, in that time, a better and more advanced musician than I was. It came as a shock, but I learnt that I couldn't afford to rest and be complacent in a world of talented and committed people with a curiosity and sense of purpose as strong as mine. These are moments of dismay and clarity which we all need if we are going to focus on anything. And in the music profession, the fact is, time does matter. And anyone serious about music, sport and dance needs those pathways from a very young age.

The reality is that state school children, or children from backgrounds and schooling that refuse competition or challenge, will find themselves in a workforce, or higher education landscape, where they will have to compete. Whether we are talking about conservatoire or university, the music industry or another career, it is a fact that auditions, interviews, performance, preparation and peril loom large. What is the effect on particular groups of young people if we expunge the art of competition from the state sector?

In the world of music scholarships and bursaries, very little can be gained without the ability to compete. Most of these critical financial benefits – often the lifeline for joining a course, playing an instrument, living and eating – are won through audition, or live competition. How, otherwise, can we decide who has potential, or has reached the necessary technical stage to cope with a course? How do we decide that this person rather than this one should be given the rare and shrinking resources available to help the next generation of musicians, or of people with valued strengths in the workplace? Giving children the chance to hone these skills goes hand-in-hand with talking about the ideal of a level playing field. And there's an irony here. A level playing field doesn't mean everyone will win, but that, in competing, everyone gets the chance to win, or to learn what it takes to win, or simply to find out, in the heat and dust of effort, what excellence is.

However, excellence is a loaded word, and music competitions, particularly at the more advanced stages of education or career, are not without controversy. I do get impatient with the idea of 'perfection' in classical music if it leads to a kind of 'competition style' of playing that errs on the side of safe flawlessness, or perfection without stumbling but also without flair.

The balance between engaging and 'perfect' playing is an important one, and the scales should not tip too far in any direction. Sometimes a competition performance can be incredibly skilful and technically advanced, but yet neither breathtaking nor brilliant. Technique encompasses the ability to use the fine tools of practised skill to ease the path to expressing something, and adjudicators have a responsibility to assess all these aspects of performance. Music is music and its job is to communicate rather than to merely display expertise. On the other hand, a flashy show of 'performance' motifs, or emotion without technical skill, also misses the point. I am very cautious, particularly, about the type of player competitions can force you to be. The pressure to conform to certain interpretations of classical pieces or composers can be driven by a powerful group of musicians and teachers who control entry to or success in various prestigious music prizes. It took me a long time to perform Bach, for example, on a public stage due to the rigidity of views of how the music should be interpreted. Fixed divisions are drawn between schools of thought, and a candidate or performer needs to brace themselves for the risk of being found on the wrong side of a vehement disagreement. Fashion often dictates what is acceptable in any field of music, and what is fashionable or deemed authentic can be controlled from a very narrow and very great height. That control has, to a certain degree, pushed Bach's music into an entire sub-genre in cello-playing, and although ubiquitous for any cello student, Bach presents a world of trepidation in competition and on the world stage.

For example, as a child I loved the violin renditions of Bach by great twentieth-century violinists like Yehudi Menuhin. I still do. I particularly loved the rich, creamy use of vibrato which gave a dreamily indulgent and tender sound to the music. Then I discovered that vibrato – or the width of vibrato and its place in the phrase – was a subject of heated debates about authenticity and style. The instruments Bach would have composed for were baroque violins and cellos, using curved bows (vaguely reminiscent of an archer's bow) with shorter hair-length and a much lighter weight at the tip where sound would diminish in wistful, airy precision. This produced a different thrill from the deep, sustained vibrato of the modern bow. Ornaments (trills or mordants – decorating the end of a phrase with oscillating notes) were more regularly used than vibrato, and vibrato itself was narrower and more subtle.

Scholarly knowledge, taste and valid discussions of interpretation all impact on how music is performed and recorded, and all of this points to a lively, healthy world of music, with which it is stimulating and necessary to engage. If I am going to call on the need for excellence, it seems impossible to ignore how that judgement is made and how it shapes the direction of higher education and professional music.

The interplay between competitions and the emphasis on digital, recorded music can be both problematic as well as full of exciting possibilities. The edited soundtrack cleaned of mistakes, or performed until mistakes are corrected, constructs an audience mindset expecting the same. Candidates tutored to win competitions take their potential professional life by the throat in that exciting, live moment of taking a risk, following insight or instinct, or relying on personal judgement. To contradict a particular competition culture, or seek to break the expected mould, is fraught with pitfalls. Alternative doors need to be kept ajar for entry to the music industry, whether within or completely outside competition success. The inclusion of the 'Audience Prize' in several big competitions can widen the possibilities for young performers but is heavy with the danger of undermining the official winner. The Audience Prize allows the competition audience to give their verdict of the most engaging or impressive candidate, regardless of the panel's decision, and is used in several major international music competitions.

Possibilities for gaining performance opportunities are small for those without influential backing or money, and that financial backing often comes with competition exposure. We need to be clear about our aims and to understand the demands of the recorded versus the live performance, and to think about what we are teaching musicians to strive for. We need to be clear about what we imagine an artist to be, or maybe that will always be determined by context and need. And if we are going to talk about excellence, we can't shrink from its implications or its ideological inequalities.

5. Relevance and Power

Some of my proudest moments are perhaps not the most obvious, or most widely known. The tributes or performances that change or move me most deeply are not necessarily the ones with the brightest halo or loudest fanfare. There have been brilliant occasions where my parents and family have shone with pride, and some that have fulfilled dreams I almost never dared to have. Playing Elgar's cello concerto at Carnegie Hall, New York, in 2022, and before that at the BBC Proms, Royal Albert Hall, London, in 2019; or Dvořák's cello concerto at the Proms in 2021, or the concertos with the New York, Los Angeles, Czech and Stockholm Philharmonics, the London Symphony, the Philharmonia, tours of East Asia, Europe, Australia, the USA, and recitals in iconic concert halls and on famous stages: there have been incredible, exciting and extraordinary concerts, collaborations and events that are now too many to list. My life has been running at an intensive speed since I won BBC Young Musician in 2016 and I am always working, travelling, practising, playing, learning and performing. It's an extraordinary life and a fascinating one. I feel, every day, that I'm doing what

I was born to do, and the cello is the instrument I was born to play.

I feel myself to be simultaneously in a place of fateful inevitability as well as one of inconceivable luck. I could not have been anything other than who I am with this drive and love of the music I play, and yet how remarkable it is that I am here. I don't question the power of the music that lives inside me, or try to over-analyse the intensity of its effect on the moods or feelings of those who listen. The reach of any music is always further and deeper than can immediately be seen, and its relevance to the lives of others unquantifiable.

I'm often moved and surprised by the smallest responses in the humblest of places from those who are the least noticed. I recently visited the brand-new Shireland CBSO Academy in West Bromwich, a state school within the Shireland Collegiate Academy Trust, headed by Sir Mark Grundy. The curriculum is immersed in music, made possible through its partnership with the City of Birmingham Symphony Orchestra. I thought back to my time at Trinity School, Nottingham, and saw the wonderful potential of this new school, emerging out of the gloom and doom of the budget cuts and attacks on state school music. As soon as I walked inside, a sense of possibilities and optimism welcomed me in. This wasn't because I was suddenly faced with a crowd of astonishingly accomplished musicians, but in front of me was the first Year 7 intake of eleven- and twelve-year-olds who had a chance to embrace music without question. A choice of musical instruments and instrument lessons was on offer to all the children, and class music lessons were spread throughout the week. Music was everywhere, in the facilities – recording equipment, concert hall, computer technology for composition and listening – and music teachers. What impressed me most was the atmosphere of gentleness and calm, and the sense of order. These were not children from homes of financial privilege in any way, and the school had been founded in a diverse metropolitan, industrial centre of the West Midlands. The children largely came from homes unconnected with classical music or with instrument-learning, and here their secondary school education would be saturated with music, with regular visits from the orchestra, and a school life very naturally and seamlessly filled with music.

After walking round the school, I had a chat and gave a performance to a small group of pupils who were learning the cello. They listened quietly and when I asked if there were any questions, they were shy and reticent in the way I'm used to when I visit state schools. Then one boy gave his reaction to the unaccompanied piece I had played. It was a growling, low and intimate piece in a minor key. He had said nothing at all during the session and I had the impression that he rarely spoke or opened up. But I could see that my playing had made a connection with him, and his face was full of emotion. 'The music was really sad,' he said.

In the months since then, I have performed to large audiences and standing ovations in great concert halls in Europe, the USA, London, and around the world, and given my heart and soul to every venue and listener. And yet, the quiet, natural, simple response of that eleven-year-old boy to my classroom cello-playing has stayed with me and given me unceasing validation.

What is the place – the relevance – of the music industry and of the musician in our world? Music is often overloaded with questions about its significance or its purpose in society. We are continually at war with what is deemed appropriate or fitting for our culture, our era or our youth. This sense of battle rages acutely over the arts, over education and in the political economics of funding. And there is so much at stake.

You can make 'relevance' mean whatever you want it to, depending on where you're standing, but the necessity of decoding the word always makes it problematic. What is relevant to one person, one group, one place is always dependent on history and emotion, or on class and geography – but indubitably on an agenda – and music is brimming with competing agendas. But I always keep in mind that quiet boy in the school classroom, or the letters I get with personal stories about how the music I play has soothed grief or helped an elderly parent. Music need not be political, and yet it often is.

What is the place – the relevance – of the music industry, and of the musician in our world? Should music be for everyone, and available to all people to consume and enjoy on a daily, or weekly basis? What is the place of music in our national culture, in the community and in the entertainment industry? And in any case, what do we mean by our 'national culture', and what is our 'community'?

Classical music is often pushed into a niche heavy with these overloaded meanings. It is lauded or accused as the representation of an elite and resolutely high culture that speaks its own, rarefied language, sitting like a fixed jewel in the rush and change of popular culture. I say lauded and accused because both its defenders and its detractors often assume the same accepted language to praise or defame it, by talking about high culture and low culture and who the imagined consumers of these cultures are. But what is high or low culture?

The idea of classical music as part of elite culture depends on particular views of its content and history. It's often seen as a historical artefact, groaning under the weight of its own illustrious heritage, to be approached with either reverence or fear. Its language is frequently seen to be elevated and difficult. The Italian, German or French words embedded in the scores of celebrated composers often need translation and it can seem accessible only to those privileged enough to be granted the keys. This leads to arguments that classical music is inherently difficult and historically exclusive, making the discussion of its relevance now a keen issue for decisions about education and provision.

But actually, classical music is both historical *and* modern, and many of its composers are very much still living. There are many traditions and genres within classical music, and room for differing tastes, different specialities and competing, vibrant paths for evolution and change. The relevance of classical music in particular, or all other types of music in general, depends on this energetic interplay between history and the present. We learn so much from the traditions and music of the past, and understand so much about the enduring power and beauty of music in the present. As with other musical styles – rap and hip-hop, for example – we are constantly paying tribute to the past. We build our sense of ourselves through this realization that we are not the first, or the best, but part of something bigger – something that will always need to be contextualized, reappraised, rediscovered and reinvented.

Education policy and funding decisions often seem caught in a circular logic, creating a situation that is then decreed as inevitable. Making music (as a subject of study, or a practical pursuit) accessible only to the privileged inevitably makes it less relevant to most people – merely because it's out of reach. Relevance, then, is a political argument.

I'm also interested in the anxiety that keeps surfacing in these discussions about relevance that classical music is a Western art form, as though this disqualifies it from wider provision. Its emergence from history as a Western art form does not rule out its relevance to those whose heritage, nationality or culture is non-Western. The astonishing strength and flowering of classical music in East Asia, particularly China and South Korea, is testament to this. The consumers and champions of classical music are not exclusively in Western countries, and neither are the producers and performers. The assumption that 'Western' excludes those in the UK whose origin, parentage or heritage is rooted in Britain's former colonial empire or beyond is based on problematic conclusions. Those of us with family ties in the diaspora of formerly colonized people, for example, are very much an integral part of Western culture. For centuries, people whose origins are non-Western have defined and continue to define the 'West'. And there are many other music genres that have emerged as Western art forms without the same weight of 'irrelevance' or non-inclusivity: rap, R&B, jazz, to name a few.

There are many arguments and historical revisions which highlight the roots of rock and roll, country, blues and many other musical forms that were always infused, inaugurated and defined by Black artists before being appropriated as mainstream music. And by mainstream, by Western, by European, by British, what do we really mean? I worry that many things are said covertly and accepted without being challenged. By Western, do we really mean White? In which case, it's important to look hard at our definitions of Western, European and British, and interrogate what we mean and who is included. Classical music is not immune to these questions, and arguments about relevance are shot through with stories and ideas that thrive on invisibility, denial and ignorance. So perhaps one task of anyone trying to champion classical music is to explore Western history itself and the place of music in the national tales we tell. And, if classical music has been co-opted by a restrictive view of our history, how do we blow that open and how much does it impact on music today?

I am continually engaged with issues around *classical* music particularly, but classical is not a separate and wholly distinct arena in the music world. Classical music is everywhere: in film and television scores, advertisements, within other styles of music, and just as popular, recognized tunes. Its boundaries are contested, politicized, and subject to an intense context of prejudice, obfuscation and fear – from without and within. My intention is to break down these perceived boundaries and to widen engagement in classical music among those who now struggle with a feeling of exclusion.

There is a range of possible approaches to this. Should

we revolutionize the *spaces* where classical music is traditionally played, or regularly remove it to new spaces? Or does the music *itself* need to change? It could be a question of information, knowledge and opportunity rather than venue and tradition. We may need, in some cases, to adapt the *culture* of classical music. But in other cases, we could just throw open the doors and welcome all people into that pre-existing culture. Many changes will arise from that, including diversifying the audiences and making them represent a wider demographic – a greater mix of young and older people, different classes and ethnicities perhaps. We need to confront the question of relevance by asking *who* we want to be the consumers and champions of this music.

What, then, is specific about classical music? In breaking down barriers we need to think deeply about the music itself and whether classical music demands something different, something special from the listener. If I stand by the importance of educating schoolchildren in music, I need to address why, and whether there is something inherent in classical music that demands a different kind of listening and a particular approach to really understand it. I need to ask whether there's a certain kind of concentration – a knowledge or an education – needed to be in the audience, and whether classical requires a particular type of attention or listening skill.

These questions apply to every type of music, but

society gets a more blanket exposure to, for example, dance music, rock, rap, and in more muted ways, jazz, and because of this, the wider public's appreciation of these genres tends to be greater, simply through exposure. The barriers to consuming many other genres of music are unequal and often perceived as non-existent. We are brought up in, and often saturated by, the language of music outside classical music, encouraged to believe we understand it as fluently as natives and that it belongs to all of us. And yet, classical is also ubiquitous, lurking in the shadows of other forms of art, television, film and video games.[1] Classical music is embedded in music clothed in another name, hiding its shame around the corners and shaded nooks of other genres, ever in translation. Because of this, it makes no sense to me that classical music is so often charged with the labels 'exclusive' or 'elitist'.

As a musician, I look for inspiration everywhere. I apply the same intensity of archival interest and 'nerdy' attention to forms of reggae, spirituals, rap, jazz and hip-hop as I do to classical. In all genres, there are echoes between styles and tracks, historical lineage and influences. All genres reward awareness of the leakages between forms, blended and corrupted origins, hacking, riffs and sampling. What we call a 'tribute' or condemn as an appropriation; what we call 'pure' or outlaw as degraded or illegitimate, are socially and culturally determined. We, of course, consume music socially and

THE POWER OF MUSIC

culturally, and all live music has its implied and understood rituals and expectations.

I was introduced to classical music as a young child in two ways. My parents played it to us at home and they also took us to concerts where we could hear the music live. These places for live classical music were churches and concert halls, and for me, it was primarily Nottingham's wonderful Royal Concert Hall where classical music lived and breathed. We were taken here on regular trips, affordable with our under-twenty-five 'Go Cards' for £5 entry, and I loved walking into the hallowed hall with tiers of seats rising above my head and the feeling of over two thousand people sharing one experience together. The concert hall performed a magic trick. Where several hundred people shuffled in and sat, shoulder-to-shoulder, knees behind heads on rising seats, and the stalls progressively sank back under the first tier in a wash of sound, I felt a paradoxical sense of great space and separateness. Isolated in the personal bubble of my own seat, people ranged around me in vast semicircles, like the regal galleries of a splendid court. It was as though we'd all gathered in anticipation of a beautiful and sacred rite.

I don't remember consciously learning the rules of being an audience member. There were no lessons and no instruction manual, no contractual terms to read and sign. I simply watched, attentive to those around me who suddenly broke into applause as the leader and then the conductor strode on to the stage and took their bows in front of the orchestra. As if under a spell, we fell silent before the first note sounded. I heard the coughing and shuffling of many bodies sighing into place and I felt that settling into consciousness of a vigilance so alert and alive it almost hurt. What was clear to me – or rather implicitly demonstrated – was the requirement for a kind of watchful listening particular to this place. The music, detailed and acoustic, was able to spill and fill the hall in all its shining threads because our concentration gave it life, and warmth and meaning. I learnt what it meant to sink into a piece of music, to really hear it, and to share that patient, open listening with a crowd of others, right there and then. The special, never-to-be-repeated singular moment of that live experience somehow grew into a space larger and more significant than its allotted time because it was collective, because it was shared, and because it was uninterrupted.

The more concerts I went to, the better I understood what I preferred, and how to distinguish one performance from another. At first, I was merely learning to separate one composer or era of music from another. I began to recognize Beethoven, Mozart, Tchaikovsky, Mahler, Shostakovich. Then I began to understand historical context and connections. And finally the orchestras, the artists, the conductors became visible to me. What were they each doing that was special to them individually? What sound were they making that was personal, or different? Why did I feel that particular way with that set of musicians or with that soloist? I now consider it a great gift that I can listen to all kinds of classical music with the freedom that experience and knowledge afford. And, crucially, what was *relevant* to me grew from repeated, familiar visits and from the rewards of listening in depth and stillness.

It's something I've only come to appreciate as an adult, but attending concerts is not unlike going to church on Sundays. At church, I was expected to be quietly attentive, and to appreciate the links between music and spirituality, between music and ritual. Music in church, through the singing of hymns or listening to a choir, or prayers sung at Mass, helped me to understand the live lineage between church and concert hall. Listening to classical music in live concerts is an intensely individual, reverential act, while at the same time being communal and ritualistic. Mass inculcated the need to stand or kneel, to be attentive to silence and to vocal, communal script. It was a similar double-consciousness of personal and collective experience, existing simultaneously with self and congregation. When I was taken to Mass as a young child, my parents tell me I spent most of each service whispering to myself as I shifted and fidgeted on the kneeler. They left me to crawl about, making up stories or acting out scenes in my head, as long as I made no noise and attracted no attention. It was fine to spend my primary years in this half-aware life, just below the surface of a comforting communion of meaning, learning almost by instinct rather than by intellect. The chants and muted singing washed over my head quite peacefully and I watched, wide-eyed, when everyone suddenly bobbed down to my eye level in genuflection.

In both spaces, I was introduced calmly and naturally. I had no idea that I was being taught to understand anything at all, and I learnt to be comfortable there merely by example. Of course, there were consequences if I did attract attention or make noise in church. The stern look from Mum or Dad that promised trouble once in the car or at home was a portent that would stop each of us in our tracks, and I regularly had to forfeit my sugar-free mint due to noisy or irritating behaviour. But, even as 'the naughty one' in the family, I never wandered out of line at concerts, sitting in my seat with every nerve alive.

The alignment of church to concert hall came with the fact that many performances of classical music took place – and still take place – in church buildings. The altar has often doubled as recital stage, either for our own performances as children and teenagers, or for watching other recitals and community orchestras. Churches are beloved of lunchtime recitals, amateur orchestras, music festivals and choirs outside and within the scope of religious ceremonies. The blurred lines between concert recital and worship originate, as well, in the actual music itself. The requiems, Masses, and the roots of so much classical music begin with the church and I grew to love the 'Amen cadence' at the same time as I understood, from music theory, the meaning of 'plagal'. When I studied the cadences for music theory, and was taught to break down what was actually taking place in the music – that a plagal cadence is, in simple terms, a move from the fourth note in the scale back to the tonic-first note – it helped me to visualize and to be conscious of how music knowledge enlarges the possibilities of music appreciation. You don't have to know the mechanics of music theory in order to love the sound and recognize the effect, but it opened up new planes of reality when I could align that effect of peaceful, almost sorrowful eternity with the mathematics of key and interval.

So, if we accept that listening and sitting quietly is a requirement in religious spaces, why does this same requirement in performance spaces make classical music exclusive? In an age where churchgoing is less ubiquitous and state schools less rigidly disciplined, should classical move with the times and release its audiences from silence? Is it the very culture of classical that bars people from its doors, struck with anxiety that they will be asked to sit still?

We need to acknowledge that there are groups of people who do feel excluded, maybe primarily for these anxieties, and that these very anxieties feed into notions of elitism and 'doing the wrong thing'. We allow for exclusivity if we deny that it exists, and our solutions depend on our diagnoses of the cause. Beyond any physical denial of access into concert halls and churches, there are practical and cultural barriers that can nonetheless feel insuperable.

As a child, I had to *learn*, by practice and example, to *listen* to the music. If we don't fling open the doors and educate children to also hear the music, if we don't explain the musical traditions, meanings and structures, if we don't demonstrate the importance of emotional engagement and the value of concentration, it makes it hard to find a way in. How can we expect children to *hear* a language we don't *teach* them? It makes the music difficult.

One of the practical barriers is the entrance to the concert hall. There are brilliant schemes run by certain concert halls and music societies across the UK that encourage children and young people through the doors by getting tickets to them. Apart from the subsidized Go Card subscription run by Nottingham's Royal Concert Hall, I remember going to watch concerts here in a party of primary school friends because the tickets were handed out in class. For most of those children it was their very first time in a concert hall and their baptism into classical music. I will never forget the reverence, the astonishment, the excitement on their faces as they watched the orchestra onstage, right in front of them, and could see the relationship between sound and instrument, the extraordinary thrill of live, acoustic music.

I have witnessed this since, in the USA, in many concerts I've been part of, and tours I've played. Recently, while playing Elgar's concerto with the Cleveland Orchestra, there were several young Black and disadvantaged teenagers who came, for the very first time, to see me and the orchestra play live. Afterwards, they came to see me backstage and seemed to be overwhelmed by the experience. I thought, then, of my own alert wonder in Nottingham's concert hall, with all my senses heightened, watching every instrument and hearing every sound. Why would we keep this revelation a secret?

We can make our traditional venues welcome to a wider group of people, without the risk of breaking our contract with silence or jeopardizing our rituals of concentration and reverence. We have to confront the tension between wanting new crowds to enter, and the worry that they will bring other behavioural expectations tied to other types of music with them. The question is, could that fracture the beautiful, tender conciliation we have with stillness?

One way in which some organizations approach this issue is to put on special performances for children and families, or tailored towards neurodiverse audiences. Sometimes these are called 'relaxed' shows, or open concerts. I have performed in several of these concerts and love, for example, seeing children move to sit closer, cross-legged on the floor, or swaying on their feet to the music. Feeling able to respond naturally and freely with no risk of censure or of annoying others is a relief for all present, and a way of keeping tradition alive side-by-side with unrestricted welcome. And perhaps our notion of 'owning' the space and the 'right' response needs sometimes to be challenged. Many venues already have to remind their traditional audiences not to cough randomly or incessantly, particularly in the quietest of moments. As well as performing at London's Wigmore Hall, I also regularly attend recitals there. An announcement always precedes the concert as the members of the audience are settled and waiting in their seats, to please try to refrain from coughing. This invariably leads to laughter and a rousing wave of immediate and irresistible coughing – but it works!

There are alternative approaches, which release classical music from the rarefied space of a concert hall, church or recital hall. I adore playing in Nottingham's Royal Concert Hall, in the perfect acoustic of Wigmore Hall, the warm sound of Liverpool's Philharmonic Hall, Boston's Jordan Hall or the Concertgebouw in Amsterdam, to name a very few. I would find it unspeakably sad to give up these engineered soundscapes, discerning audiences and the weight of knowledge, appreciation or history these places hold. Likewise, I am inspired by the beauty of sound in so many other concert and recital halls: New York's Carnegie Hall, Vienna's Musikverein, the Berliner Philharmonie, the Elbphilharmonie in Hamburg, Lucerne's or Stockholm's concert halls. These were all built in glorious honour and understanding of classical music in a way that a theatre, school hall or gig venue has not been. I want to challenge and be challenged by the vast experience and knowledge of audiences who are deeply in love with classical music and who have sat through concerts and recitals of the greatest artists through decades, as well as play to those who have studied or worked at the art of music for most of their young lives. I want to listen, myself in the audience, to my peers, mentors and predecessors who demonstrate for me the fascinating interplay of great musicians with wonderful hall with attentive audience, and the sorcery that fosters. I was wooed and romanced into these places and learnt my art in order to be part of them, longing to be worthy and longing to be heard.

But I also long to be heard by those people who halt at the doors of these places and refuse the music because they either refuse or fear the culture they perceive to be lurking within. My mother used to say, when I came home from school, that I needed to learn to be bilingual – there was a language for friends and a language for home, and a different lexicon was required in each circumstance. And I carry that cultural bilingualism with me still, knowing by instinct or practice – as we all do – what language we should use in which context. And we're not talking about a different language altogether but a shift in style, perhaps, or emphasis, or physical gestures or vocabulary to suit a location. Music is a language of many dialects, but the language essentially remains the same.

There are several projects that work to bring a different audience to classical music by changing the venue, and even by challenging the nature of 'venue'. My siblings and I have played several times, either as recital soloists, chamber artists or concerto soloists in the multistorey car park venue close to Peckham Rye overground station in London. This is home to the 'Bold Tendencies' series, and it is where my sister Jeneba played Rachmaninov's Piano Concerto No. 2 with the Philharmonia Orchestra; where Isata and I, together and separately, have played solo recitals and chamber concerts; and where we all, as a family, have performed together. This performance space is a floor of the car park, with great concrete slabs and pillars holding up a concrete roof and one side open to a clear, wide overview of the populous, built-up cityscape. On the street outside is a bustling, vibrant, multicultural community, and I arrive from the station, cello on my back, and walk past stalls selling plantains, hot peppers and jollof rice, hearing the Krio of my mum's childhood being spoken, and knowing that the audience inside the venue will look quite different to most concert-hall clientele. I clamber up the cement-hard steps to the top of the car park, spread out to the sky, where the London summer or early autumn brings glorious red twilight over the sprawling landscape all around us; and during the concert on the lit-up floor below, trains thunder and whistle underneath at rumbling, shaking intervals.

The stunning success of this series of concerts attests to the fact that there are real gains to be made from turning unlikely and unromantic venues, not originally sanctified for classical use, into forums that therefore belong to everyone. And notwithstanding the change of audience, or the regular cacophony of the underground, or the gently seasonal air coming in with the sunset, that beautiful, meditative concentration still settles and softens all around us. Everyone is listening, everyone is watching and everyone understands what the music requires, both those who do regularly attend classical concerts and those who do not. And perhaps that's because there is a mix of both.

Another initiative which has had resounding success is 'Through the Noise'. This runs crowdfunded gigs for classical music, and in their 'Noise Nights', classical musicians perform in venues ordinarily home to other music genres. Gone is the seating, tiered or otherwise, and in its place audience members stand, as closely as they can jostle together, to watch and listen to the musicians onstage. The gigs are shorter in length – one hour rather than two halves with an interval – and the cheers and shows of appreciation tend to be louder, drinks in hand, and in keeping with the venues' mostly younger audience members. I've played many times with this series and so have my brother and sisters, and we love the freedom it gives us to mix classical with jazz or folk music or improvisation.

These gigs have the effect of implicitly melting the borders between genres and easing the perceived orthodoxy of classical music, and yet the listening and the concentration are still there. The shift from 'concert' to 'gig' in the naming of these performances is important because the usual characteristics of what we mean by a concert are loosened and shifted. Perhaps the listening is more open, without preconceptions and unworried by conformity. Perhaps the music is speaking another dialect here, possessing a new freedom and a mutated, changed meaning. Or perhaps we have just presented it to a wider range of people who understand it – released from context – in just the same way. When my brother, Braimah, with our friend Plínio Fernandes, the Brazilian guitarist, toured with Through the Noise and played a concert at the Rescue Rooms in Nottingham, I was in the audience, having grown up with this iconic gig venue for non-acoustic bands. It was a night I'll never forget. The sold-out space was full of people I'd been at school with, people who'd taught me at school, my neighbours – older and younger – and people from all generations and interests and backgrounds. It was a groundswell response to Through the Noise bringing classical music to a wider audience – laying bare its links with folk, South American and European music, tango and jazz, while also playing Paganini and Bach's Partitas. An atmosphere of elated generosity charged the room and it felt like rejoicing.

It's clear that, when we make decisions about performance venues and plans, we need to think first about who we are trying to reach. The power and relevance of any art form and any music is determined by its consumers, and classical music risks redundancy if we separate it entirely into discrete, closed and jealously guarded spaces. Of course, there is more to this than the venue, but we bring people in if we first go out and find them. The act of keeping classical music away from the general public, from those without private education or a certain kind of cultural acumen, serves to exclude and marginalize the music itself. Every engagement with the arts is a cultural engagement, but our individual experiences with culture – and, accordingly, how confident we feel in the spaces where we consume culture – comes from the education we receive, the families and places we grow up in, the social classes we belong to. Culture is something that can be acquired.

And if the general public do come into concert and recital halls, and they break our passionately held traditions, what then? One particularly common contentious issue is the phenomenon of 'not clapping between movements' of a concerto or sonata. This is one of the conventions of classical music, learnt the hard way by my mother, who had never been to a concert hall until she took us as children, and found herself clapping with no one else joining in. A classical symphony, concerto or sonata typically has three or four movements, and the applause is traditionally reserved for after the last movement and not in between them. This is a learnt tradition because every movement has a recognizable end – the resolution of a theme or a mood, followed by a gap and a pause – and it is this moment of silence into which the inexperienced members of an audience, like my mother at her first concerts, find it obvious and natural to clap, breaking the unwritten rule. When it has happened during my performances, which it has on many occasions, it only makes me happy. This is not disrespect or willed ignorance but a desire to show appreciation and give back to the performer. The transgression is not an active rudeness but a lack of awareness of what is, in fact, a relatively recent practice. It has not always been the done thing *not* to clap, and when it happens it tells me that there are people listening who do not normally attend classical music concerts – but here they are.

In this frightening age of concert halls being closed due to the withdrawal of funds, we need to stand up for our recital spaces in the same way we would stand up for our cathedrals. They were built in the service of the music – the particular music – they are designed to deliver. Classical music – in the form of orchestras, or chamber ensembles, or choirs, or solo concerts – has inspired buildings and rooms specifically designed and acoustically engineered to empower life and soul and sound. The tiered seats, or the position of the seating, the shape of the ceiling, the building materials – all are formed with the deliberate love and knowledge that emerge from music meeting science, and all is made possible and sustainable by economic and societal choices. I'm thinking, painfully, of Wales's national concert hall, St David's Hall in Cardiff. This beautiful, purpose-built hall, beloved of orchestras and chamber musicians alike, has been subject to ongoing threats of closure for a few years. The first announcement by the council was a desire to rip out the tiered seating and re-purpose the space for non-acoustic gigs, making it no longer primarily a hall for classical music. Since this announcement, it was declared that the hall would close permanently, and the news was met with protests from the classical music world. Following this, the council has claimed that St David's Hall is in urgent need of repair and has closed it until further notice.

I feel pessimistic about my chances of ever again being able to enter this hall in which I and all my siblings have performed at various times over the years. It would be an unspeakable loss. As we risk losing opportunities for children to learn music, we are also losing our dedicated homes of classical music, and like churches of different denominations or faiths, we need to retain our rich range of choices.

In fact, it's a very long time since the home of classical music was exclusively the concert hall. It's also been the recording, or the dedicated radio channel. In earlier days of television and radio, and in the not-so-distant past, it lived happily on prime-time television and its classical stars were the stuff of popular imagination. For my parents' generation, watching stars like Julian Lloyd Webber, André Previn, James Galway or Nigel Kennedy on television was neither niche nor unusual. But the fact is, these musicians were listened to because they had airtime, and the decline of classical music on popular media is due not so much to a public dislike as to an echoing lack of visibility. Those in charge of programming have expunged classical out of mainstream and prime television slots and tidied it away into corners dealing exclusively with 'the arts', or 'education', or 'special interest.'

Social media platforms are now crucial to the dissemination of classical music and the musicians who play it. Our own Facebook Lives during lockdown, for example, gained more viewers than a long-running concert tour could have achieved, and classical stars such as Nicola Benedetti, Anna Lapwood, Jess Gillam and Hilary Hahn, for example, use their social media platforms to sell out their concert spaces. And, of course, there are exceptions to the decline of classical music stars on television, with Lang Lang's incredibly popular appearances on Channel 4's *The Piano*, gaining record viewing figures.

When I won BBC Young Musician in 2016, the programme was already in choppy waters. Since 1978, the competition had been transmitted in full, every performance programme of each competitor from the Category Finals onwards included in their entirety. My parents spent their childhood and teens watching hours of recitals and concertos by other teenagers, along with the vast majority of television viewers in the UK. The winners were national celebrities, and the competition launched stellar classical careers. The programme carried with it an air of mystique and romance so powerful that an entire generation of British musicians dreamt of their time onscreen, playing to an audience of millions and fantasizing the applause received for the hours and hours of practice they had put in. By the time I – and my brother and sisters – were deep in this seductive dream scenario, the BBC were cutting its airtime and moving it away from the main channels. BBC Young Musician was fast becoming 'special interest' because of its reduced availability. Apparently, audiences no longer had the attention span for full category recitals, and the category and semi-final results, already decided on recorded reels, determined the content of clips and commentary.

Even so, a substantial amount of content was aired,

the advertising was as energetic as ever, and the final concertos were broadcast in full. My fellow finalists – the saxophonist Jess Gillam, and the French-horn player Ben Goldscheider – and I were given our chance to show our concertos from beginning to end, with no edits or cuts to the televised version. In this way, the cameras could reveal what this all meant in terms of preparation, practice and the impact on our families. The full concertos we performed on the day had taken weeks or even a year of our time, love and effort. I had spent my childhood watching with wonder as those not much older than me demonstrated the rewards of incredible hard work, commitment and sheer, deep love of an art form for which they put themselves on the line. All this was available to me, easily on terrestrial television, shared with a general public that valued this. I was inspired, stimulated, seduced and given hope to pursue something that demanded passion and self-belief, confidence and effort. And even more than this, I was encouraged to create something beautiful. The shift to social media and to streaming is inevitable and offers new possibilities. The challenge now is to not lose hold of the avenues for young musicians that worked so well, or to replace them with new outlets and dedicated exposure.

The Covid-19 pandemic and subsequent recession have arguably accelerated the way our national broadcasting media is turning a cold shoulder to music-learning and inspiration. The UK is trying to emerge from the ruins of a pandemic that ravaged our economy and particularly our arts institutions. The elephant-in-the-room, rampaging at will, is Brexit, which has isolated the music industry in general from the rest of Europe, stranding musicians, orchestras and bands on an island squeezed of funding and stoked into panic. The additional costs and administrative requirements for British musicians to travel to perform in Europe have made it impossible for many players and orchestras to do so. British musicians have also become far less attractive to European organizers who have to pay a great deal more for their presence and wade through a lot of paperwork. Those most affected are up-and-coming young musicians, trying to develop their careers, as well as orchestras, bands and chamber music groups whose costs are multiplied by their numbers. In a statement on BBC Radio 3's programme *Music Matters*, former BBC Young Musician winner and world-renowned violinist Nicola Benedetti summed up the isolation of the British music industry by saying: 'We have a level of perfect storm that is not mirrored across Europe. The combination of post-Covid and Brexit is disastrous on so many levels.'[2]

Like other classical music broadcasting, coverage of the BBC Young Musician competition is becoming a side issue, dropping out of view for a public that is largely offered only quick-fix light entertainment and unthreatening familiarity, even though what is familiar is precisely a consequence of what is provided. And if a regular television viewer is denied the consumption of a full-length, unedited and uninterrupted concerto, they won't know they want it. I'm not sure social media can bridge this gap, relying as it does on shorter, more immediately exciting content. It has become more difficult to emerge from the shadows if you are a young musician with nothing but hard work, dedication and love to spur you into the hope of recognition and a career. Of course, it takes far more than television to make a musician, but the survival of any art form depends largely on the glamour and pervasiveness of its marketing, and perhaps that's part of the issue. In a changing media landscape, the marketing of classical music needs to adapt and keep up. Perhaps marketing is the key to classical music's chance of relevance.

But what are we trying to make music relevant to? Ever since the Council for the Encouragement of Music in the Arts was set up in 1940, with an explicit goal of promoting and developing a sense of Britishness, arts funding has never been absent from political battles. Funding for creative industries is regularly accused of elitism or bias, controlled or restrained by tactical funding decisions or dramatic budget reductions. Arts Council England's launch of 'Let's Create' in 2020 sought to scatter the funding concentration in London to areas outside the capital, controversially starving a world-class centre for music, including internationally renowned arts institutions, in a stated mission to decentralize. The idea of spreading funding outside London is laudable if it leads to extra money, yet the proposed ransacking of excellence at the centre, removing funding from internationally celebrated temples of music, opera, theatre and ballet, seems to go directly against the arts. The idea is to strip support from areas of privilege and redirect it to the grass-roots, struggling, more amateur and less developed projects and regions that serve more local or particular needs. Unfortunately, the local environment across the UK is battling stringent cuts to council funding, with councils like Birmingham and Nottingham City going bankrupt. Without a thriving local landscape for music, we are planting unsupported seeds in random fashion and building a system that pits one arts institution against another.

The problem here is similar to the prime-time television purge. Once there is no beacon place or example of excellence for music and the arts, once you remove the shining goal and destination for young artists to aspire to, emulate and learn from, or for the public to enjoy, the light dims everywhere. As the director of Wigmore Hall, John Gilhooly, stated on BBC Radio 4, addressing accusations of elitism aimed at prestigious music venues: 'This isn't about being elitist. These are elite musicians. There's a huge difference. They're like Olympic athletes. They train for years, for decades to perfect their art and they need these great platforms. And we shouldn't be diluting the quality of what they're offering us at any cost.'[3]

The attitude of any government to its arts sector reflects the society and the ideological battles of the time, and music is right at the centre of this. I think now of the Chechen Republic's government decree in April 2024, which bans any music faster than 116 beats per minute and slower than 80 beats.[4] This makes no logical sense until it's understood that most 'Western' music falls outside this permissible range, particularly the fast dance music of LGBTQ communities, damned along with musical culture from 'other' peoples, and supposedly invidious to the morality and ethics of Chechen life. The Chechen leader, Ramzan Kadyrov, was quoted as saying: 'Borrowing musical culture from other peoples is inadmissible.'[5] Music is often forced into 'relevance' to the state ideology that funds it and gives it bandwidth, or the state chooses the kind of music that suits its claims of equity, or cultural purity, or history, or ethics. Relevance can often be translated into convenience, or conformity or expedience. Or maybe it's more accurate to state that relevance is determined by power.

We need to ask the question: Who is speaking? Who is playing music and who for? The mission statement of Arts Council England is: 'Great art and culture for everyone'. I have no idea what this really means as it says everything and nothing at the same time. Each word has to be interrogated, and each is dependent on who you are and what your mission is – which is paradoxically not explained in this mission statement. 'Great' can be a word as anodyne and empty of substance as 'nice', useful for lazy texts or for refusing to be pinned down. What is great art, and are we talking about elevated and world-class, or just fun and good? Culture can cover anything from ethnicity and geography to 'high' and 'low' art, to artistic expression. And what about 'everyone'? Does 'everyone' get a tiny bit of watered-down run-off in the effort to spread out the funds, or do we mean access to something already there? Does everyone get the chance to actually create this great art or is culture something ready-made and sanctioned? These become urgent questions when funding is tied to government whims and whimsy, or when states harden into autocracy and nationalist dictates. But interrogating the role of music and the arts in any society is always necessary, and the answers to these questions are ever reflective of the world we live in. Often, what these enquiries reflect are serious and sometimes terrifying edicts on the role of power over art, and what may seem unimportant or frivolous can reflect a wider and more sinister political will. Even if we don't get as far as terrifying or sinister, there are very real implications in these dictates about who gets to practise, consume and define the arts.

Classical music is continually having to answer questions about its relevance by finding ways to justify its public funding. Arts Council England adds tight strings to its support, demanding lengthy and time-consuming reports on contributions to local communities, education and outreach, and proof of links outside London or with disadvantaged communities. These are all emphases I champion, but not to the detriment of the music or towards the loss of elite orchestras and musicians on elite stages in the great concert and recital halls. I use 'elite' here in the way we are still allowed to use it in sport.[6] When the Olympics are broadcast for the world, or when the winner of the London Marathon crosses the finish line, nobody criticizes the use of 'elite' to describe these athletes: that is what they are. We need to be able to describe 'elite' musicians as such, without fear of complaint. And 'great' here means that there has to be a recognition of international standards of excellence in the arts at the same time that we encourage the grass roots, the amateur and the young.

The delegation of the job of music education, inclusion and access entirely to the music industry strikes me as extraordinary in a climate that sees music education stripped from schools and the disappearance of funding for local arts projects, theatres, choirs, orchestras and venues. Regional city councils, bankrupt or teetering on the edge due to slashed budgets from central government, are forced to cut music and arts funding from schools and communities at the same time that Arts Council England's 'Let's Create' insists that those who provide music performances themselves somehow fill those gaps.

Classical music thrives when both the roots and branches are given the energy and nourishment they need. Neither the water nor the sun can do the whole job alone and each does not perform the same function. Before I was ready to enter BBC Young Musician, my training came, not just through private teaching, schools, music festivals and being taken to concerts, but also through the thriving network of community and non-professional orchestras, male-voice choirs, regional orchestras and music societies which arranged local concerts and recitals. There are many unsung heroes who work tirelessly for the love of music and the desire to participate, improve and share that love with others. These groups and organizations were invaluable to me and my family, giving us opportunities to perform and practise our music skills in front of audiences when we were still very young. Full of excitement, nerves and only nascent expertise, we were able to play our instruments in 'proper' adult concerts in front of real, ticket-holding audiences and learn our craft by doing it.

My very first concerto experience came with an offer from Djanogly Community Orchestra. As a prize for winning Nottingham Young Musician on my seven-eighth-size cello, at the age of twelve, I was asked to perform Haydn's Cello Concerto No. 1 in C. By the date of the performance I was thirteen years old and still small next to the full-size cello that was being loaned to me, simply out of kindness, by a man named Frank White, who had made it himself from the perfect piece of wood he'd sourced and crafted, and to whom I had been introduced by Sarah, my cello teacher. Frank heard me play a string quartet with Braimah and Konya on violin, and Isata on viola, in a local leisure centre in the winter, the ceiling panels deadening the sound but not our enthusiasm. Full of interest, Frank let us borrow and play a full quartet of beautiful instruments he had made himself, for as long as we needed to. This gift, and others in our lives, has been an essential and shining element of the story of how I was able to become a musician. I was probably not sharply conscious then of all that had contributed to getting me there backstage, all the interconnected organizations and individuals who cared about music and cared about giving young musicians a helping hand.

My left hand held the fingerboard of the cello while my right played with the frog of the bow, absent-mindedly fantasizing that I was practising the twirling and manipulation of a fencing sword before a duel. I didn't know this was strengthening my fingers and moulding suppleness into my wrist, or that this walk on to the concerto stage would be the first of many. I was overwhelmed by the significance of the present and of what was to come.

This moment was a hugely important step in my training as a concert soloist. In order to get this opportunity, I had had to work hard to be seen and heard – to win an important, advanced, local competition and now, having been selected and given this chance, I had to prove that I was worth it.

The concert was held in St Mark's Church in Woodthorpe, Nottingham, a large, modern, Anglican church with a bright rectangular space, and I knew from the rehearsal that there would be row after row of chairs down the length of the aisle in front of the orchestra. I also knew my family would be there, right near the front, as well as Frank and his wife, Elizabeth, but I don't remember wondering or worrying whether anyone else would turn up. I had sat alone in the warm-up room at the top end, hidden from the stage, staring at the orchestra's empty instrument cases, discarded half-open or on their sides on the chairs and carpet, and listening to the players tune and warm up. I heard what sounded like a lot of clapping as the conductor, John Rayfield, walked on and began introducing the evening. I could hear them playing the first piece, but I was distracted, focusing on the first notes of the Haydn concerto and beginning to mime with bow and fingers so that my inner music was soon louder for me than the orchestra. Then, with a jolt to my thoughts, John Rayfield was in front of me, smiling and gesturing for me to follow him out in front of the waiting musicians and the waiting public.

That first, long walk with a conductor to stand and face an orchestra and audience is always heavy with anticipation. The shocking, sudden transition from backstage solipsism into a roaring spotlight of applause is always surreal and feels like an explosion too shattering to bear. This calls for a swift pulling together of the senses and driving myself into the hard, bright present of the music that's already sounding from the string section to the right and left behind me, the cellos and double basses helping to ground and stabilize me, while the violins lift and march me into the piece.

I remember looking straight at my family sitting in front of me to my left, and especially my dad, who was a full, steady presence, both benign and expectant, a call to attention and a checkpoint to which my eyes kept returning. I now rely on this fixing of significant people in the audience either before or while I play. Family members are focal points, as are friends and certainly teachers. As a performer, I need to play to everyone in the audience, and those who know, intimately, the effort and the emotional detail in what I play are like brilliant points of light. The concerto soloist sits or stands so close to the orchestra they are both inside and in front of it, surrounded and saturated within its chorus but having to thrust themselves ahead in a show of unabated conviction. But there are rules, and the greatest thing I learnt that night was the art of unremitting, universal listening and staying awake to everything around me. If I broke away from my unblinking awareness of the conductor, or forgot to pay attention to the orchestra who couldn't always second-guess my lunges and inspirations, I had to quickly rein myself in and blend my playing with their tempo.

That balance of ecstatic interpretation with strict collaboration was an art I began learning then, at thirteen, because Nottingham and the East Midlands were alive with amateur orchestras and community music societies and individuals who, at grass-roots level, cared about the future of music-making at all stages. This is a situation we all hope can continue and thrive. I had already watched Isata play Haydn's Piano Concerto in D with the same orchestra, having won the same competition a few years earlier, and my brother and all my sisters played their first concertos with Djanogly. There is still an online video of me as that child walking with the awkward gait of a new teenager with my cello to the front of the orchestra, bowing and switching my gaze repeatedly to my dad in the front row. I also hear that burgeoning love of song and telling my story the way I hear it in the moment through my cello, utterly dependent on orchestra, conductor and audience in a way that can only be fully appreciated by doing it. The church is full with family and friends of the orchestra and with people who come to hear music in their local church. It's neither grand nor elite, but simply great.

I've recently read the testament of one of the orchestra

members, Jo Bucklow, a flautist who has been with Djanogly Orchestra since its inauguration in 1988, and it sums up why we need to cherish our community music and how interrelated each individual and collective initiative is. The existence of a living, healthy network of music-making, competitions, generosity, tradition and partnerships with schools, teachers and children is what keeps music alive. As Jo says: 'This orchestra has been responsible for getting many people back to playing, not just me. This has stimulated the local music industry. Like many other players I've had occasional lessons and bought a new instrument, and attended summer schools as a result of the orchestra.'[7]

We have no hope of keeping our orchestras, our music and our music industry 'relevant' if it is made up of one particular group of people from one part of society. Enabling heterogeneity begins in different places. If we aim to increase access to something worthwhile, we can't expect every aspect of music and every institution to perform the same function – or to perform it without financial backing. A local orchestra is about the joy of 'having a go' and giving everyone a chance to participate and improve. An internationally acclaimed orchestra acts as a career pinnacle for professionals and provides music performance and interpretation at its technical best. We are talking about different, although interconnected, things when we invoke 'local', 'national' and 'international'. We all need access to all of them, and we dismantle them all by demanding the loss of one aspect in favour of another. We need to recognize the value of open rehearsals, outreach and education *alongside* excellence. I want to keep both diversity and excellence – and I demand both. I want access to both.

The concept of relevance rests in what stories we wish to tell, and whose voices we wish to hear. Where will the change, the vibrancy, the restless, exciting imagination of our music come from if we are doing nothing more than talking to ourselves in monotonous echo chambers? Diversity, in all its kaleidoscopic disruption, is necessary for the music industry to survive and to flourish. But true diversity and inclusion allows the opportunity to enjoy and to achieve excellence.

If I'm talking about the power and relevance of classical music, I can't do that without discussing the music itself. I chose to become a classical musician because of my love of the music, and its hold on me has grown and deepened every day and year since infancy. My life is defined by the music I listen to and play, and I would no longer make sense of myself without it. I express my emotions and much of my personality through music. It is how I articulate hope, joy, despair and defiance. Music is the language in which I am most fluent and through which I connect most fully with others.

The first concerto that caught my imagination, and which I wanted, desperately, to play was Elgar's Cello Concerto in E Minor. I had an immediately powerful

emotional connection with the music, and I was responding to two things. One was the passion and persuasiveness
of Jacqueline du Pré's playing, and the other was the
music itself. It was a subliminal response which I couldn't
and wouldn't have wanted to put into words. The feeling,
and the longing to transmit that feeling through my cello,
became a turbulent need in me. But I didn't yet, at the age
of six or seven, have the technical skills to achieve this
with my quarter-size cello, even though I tried and tried.
Understanding music is intensely personal and private,
but is also dependent on our connection to others. It was
Jacqueline du Pré who brought the piece to me, and then
other recordings and live experiences, as well as my grap-
plings with the notes and score over the years.

Later, I read about its context and history, about who
Elgar was, both as a historical figure and as an individual
with a personal history. I thought about his relationship
with the First World War and the loss of his son during
it, his inability to compose while he could hear the thud-
ding of artillery from his Sussex cottage, and the illness
and death of his wife in the war's aftermath. Out of
all this, wreathed in shadows of shock and grief, rises
Elgar's last major work, the cello concerto.

How much we ascribe known autobiographical detail
or assumptions about experience to the meaning of a
composition is debatable, but this can sometimes increase
our identification with the music itself. Elgar has been
repeatedly appropriated as a symbol of a particular kind

of nationalist Englishness, the kind that triumphs in the victory of war, the pomp and circumstance of battle and pride. But I don't hear that in the music. Perhaps Elgar's awkward role play as moustachioed English gentleman in tweed, emerging from a more humble childhood (with a church organist father who also tuned pianos) is there in the quiet brooding of his composition. He was self-taught, non-academic, Catholic and very much an outsider from the Englishness he later came to represent, and any notions of imperialism were adopted in middle age.

Does any of this matter to my relationship with the music? I rely on what I hear, and knowledge, whether autobiographical, contextual or musical, determines my intellectual engagement with what I play. There is no escaping the context in which I find myself – but I can transcend it – and I am deeply interested in where music comes from, its consumption then and now, and where it finds itself in different places and times. Elgar's sorrow and discomfort move me over time in a way that his supposed vaunting imperialism does not. I interpret the broken lament, the blasted requiem of the cello concerto, its devastating enquiry into human failure and cruelty, as much more relevant to me. And that's not because I have lived through war, or suffered irretrievable loss, but because empathy lives and radiates from the depths of the score.

Whenever I think about relevance, I remind myself why I am a musician. There are fundamental questions I ask myself, and convictions I hold that are greater than the sifting, sinking sands of partisan politics, or class prejudice, or cultural anxiety. I know the power of music and its relevance lies not in the stories someone else is telling about us, or the spurious barriers put in our way, but in those personal, direct moments of actually listening. In that West Midlands classroom at the CBSO academy in the summer of 2024, there was no politician, or preconception, or grand door between my cello and the pupils in front of me. None of those eleven- and twelve-year-olds cared or maybe even knew I was playing 'classical' music, because it was just music. The response was clear, emotional and sincere, and therefore, utterly relevant: 'The music is sad.'

6. Music and Identity

I was born in Bahrain, on the Persian Gulf, but grew up from the age of two in Nottingham, where Isata had been born. My mother was born in Sierra Leone and my father is the son of immigrant Caribbean parents who subsequently went back to Antigua. Some of my earliest memories are rushing headlong after a football with my sister and brother ahead of me, and dancing to 50 Cent by the dining table. I love fried plantains and Johnny cakes. I love Haydn's string quartets, Mozart, Bob Marley and recordings of Pablo Casals playing Bach. I went to school with children from African, Caribbean, Irish, Asian and English working-class and middle-class backgrounds. I supported Nottingham Forest, I watched West Indies cricket and England football, and now I support Arsenal, love most sports and go to as many concerts, plays, films, ballets and shows as I can.

I speak from several overlapping positions as an international soloist; a British classical musician; a Black, state-educated person in the arts; and an African-Caribbean man with added Welsh heritage and a complicated location within Englishness. And that's OK. Most of the time.

I find debates about national identity both poignant

and complicated. Britishness is a shifting concept and Englishness fraught and flawed. And I find myself resisting, constantly redefining or just not fitting into available concepts of national or cultural identity.

In May 2016, I became the first Black winner of BBC Young Musician since the competition began in 1978. From childhood, I would walk into concert halls and classical music recitals with my family and we would be the only Black people in the room. I knew to expect that at every music festival, residential music course, or competition the only Black children or teenagers there would be us. At the Saturday Primary and Junior Academy we were novelties or in an extreme minority.

We were all hyper-aware of this, even though it wasn't a big topic of conversation when we were small children. We were encouraged by our parents not to let this fact make us feel that we were not good enough to be there. This was an act of defiance and courage that I increasingly began to appreciate as I grew older and for which I have never stopped being grateful. The cost of walking into an audience where you are not expected can only be understood by the person who is in those shoes. To walk onstage holding a classical instrument in a room where there is no one else who looks like you, is a rebellious act. For a child in that situation, it can take its toll. The energy it takes to defend your psyche from the constant need to prove yourself against the odds puts a child at a great disadvantage and the cost can be too great.

In order to succeed in classical music, work ethic is critical. If you do not put the hours in, you cannot pass a music exam, or learn a concerto, or enter a conservatoire, or reach even the most basic rung of a career. At every stage and age the practice requirements steepen. I had to find ways to lengthen the days in order to fit in the scales, exercises, studies and memory-training that the music dictates. I had to train myself in resilience and endurance, to dedicate myself to the voice I was developing and the style I strove to achieve. I listened hard to my teachers, studied humility and screwed my courage into repetition, effort and ambition. All the while, I was taught to meditate on musicality and dig deep to find the full, confident well of my own sound.

What happens when all of that bumps up endlessly against a world that tells you, aggressively, who you are and should be? It's immensely difficult to convey to others the effect of negative stereotyping and cynicism on those who grow up in the midst of this, no matter how positive and determinedly expectant your family is, no matter how supportive your teachers and friends. Hard work and commitment need confidence and self-belief to feed on, a sure knowledge that possibilities are ahead and opportunities ready. Keeping up the force and spirit to forge on in a pursuit that takes every ounce of mental, physical and emotional energy is an existential daily struggle if we are also pushed to defend our very right to be here.

Is it fair to put Black children in this situation and ask them somehow to sort it out and get on with it? Wouldn't it be kinder to say: 'This space is not for you' rather than throw them, head-on, into an impossible corner, both psychological and practical? My family of seven siblings haven't just got on with it, but we have been resolutely and comprehensively supported by a tight network of family – parents, aunties and uncles, grandparents and cousins. We've been held up by the communities we grew up in and by the background communities of our parents and grandparents. We've had dedicated teachers and friends, and critically, we have had – and still have every day – each other.

Most of us in this category of 'Black classical musicians', that we would rather were not a category at all, keep our heads down and work daily to prove ourselves, bull-headed against the storm. Survival is in the supremacy of our art and the impeccable finesse of our technique. If we don't sing more beautifully than anyone, we will be accused of singing badly or not at all. And the more visible we are – the more vocal we become – the louder the storm against us.

When I won BBC Young Musician, I couldn't believe it had happened. When I heard my name follow Dobrinka Tabakova's much anticipated '. . . and the winner is . . .', my whole body shone with delight. My hand covered my open mouth and, as I saw when I watched the footage back later, relief mixed with impossible joy on my face. I walked out in front of the standing crowd like a boy in a dreamworld, through the looking glass into a world topsy-turvy with an incredible truth, my family in a row, crying.

I found out, much later, that social media, although mostly delighted, was also hosting a thread of darkened disbelief, turning on the idea that being Black meant I couldn't possibly have been good enough. Surely, they said, this was a 'politically correct' decision. He only won *because* he was Black. I was the first and therefore the unconscionable, impossible winner. If there were none before me, that itself was proof there should be none of us now. We were damned if we won and damned if we didn't.

Luckily, my parents folded all of this into their quiet whispering together and hid it from me. I was flushed with the happiness and the weight of winning, pressed into learning the Schumann concerto from scratch to memory in six weeks for a performance because the exigencies of the competition had allowed for no pockets of time beforehand. It was enough to win the competition as a cellist and deal with the consequences, and that task had taken all my strength.

I was very aware, though, of the kind of scrutiny I was weathering. The radio and newspaper interviews let me know without hiding it that I had questions to answer. On the one hand, was I a bona fide good cellist or 'just' a Black musician? Was I really fit to be pushed into this spotlight and stand next to 'real' classical musicians who looked authentic? On the other hand, I was challenged, without having said a thing, for making my Black identity visible and meaningful when, surely, nothing mattered but the music? I remember thinking: 'Well, clearly it's on your mind because that's what you're asking me about.' This double-bind thrust upon me of denial and yet responsibility for my identity was a confusing but familiar message, and I knew my job was to remain quiet, firm and thoughtful. The only route was working harder.

I remember, as an example, one of my first national radio interviews after winning the BBC competition. I was seventeen, and very much a teenager, with no experience of the media beyond having the odd photo taken for the *Nottingham Post*. I thought I would be talking about the concerto – Shostakovich 1 – that I had played in the final, or my relationship with the cello and music. But I found myself being grilled rather sharply on why it mattered that I was Black, and shouldn't that be an insignificant and unmentioned fact? Shouldn't Black musicians be aspiring to integrate into the mainstream without making a song-and-dance about it? I answered from a well of calm and thoughtfulness, sifting through the surface of the questions without engaging with the assumptions underneath. I remember feeling very clear about the gulf of understanding between us, and somehow already knowing it was best not to try to address this in any way. I would talk about the music, and not talk about whether or not my being Black – a fact I hadn't brought up – was an issue I should ignore.

I wanted, first and foremost, to concentrate on playing the cello, on improving all the time and being the best musician I could be. But I carried a responsibility I couldn't shake. I wanted to represent hope and possibility for children, families and people who relied on the visible fact of who I was. Having a choice didn't come into it as there was none and never had been. I couldn't pretend to be anyone I wasn't but somehow, I had to place Black and classical next to each other in a way that made perfect, undeniable and glorious sense.

In the summer of 2020, I was involved in a discussion on Zoom with other artists in the music industry about the position of Black musicians. This was the year of George Floyd's murder by police in Minneapolis and the rise in Black Lives Matter protests. We had taken to the streets as a family, struck down with the anguish that hit us all and needing the togetherness of those who understood and grieved too. This was another example out of so many when we understood that one of us represented us all, in a reality where individuality and selfhood as Black people was hard-won and often lost.

This reality was something we were all familiar with. It had been true, for example, when Braimah went on a post-A levels holiday with two friends to Spain. One of his friends was White and the other Black. At check-in, the attendant couldn't distinguish between the two Black passengers, continually mixing them up in a comedy of errors. In the end, only one of their suitcases found its destination as Braimah and his friend seemed to have become one person, interchangeable from each other. This would have been amusing if the two friends had not had to spend a week sharing the same suitcase. This anecdote has become part of our family lore, and it's one we tell with humour and ironic laughter, but it's also just one illustration of how we all cope with situations like this where we come up against our own hyper-visibility and yet individual invisibility.

The discussion we had as Black artists was how to protect Black musicians from exploitation and domination in an industry that had very few, if any, Black artist-managers, event and programme managers, staff or directors on the recording labels, or Black decision-makers and scouts. What we had to say as artists and how we wanted to say it was ringed with trepidation, and maybe opening up paths of communication between us promised a measure of protection.

There were many important arguments being made and points defended, and I agreed with a lot of them, but the group was made up of mainly non-classical Black artists – in fact, overwhelmingly so. The conversation turned on the preservation of Black music itself from exploitation and domination. But what does that mean for a Black classical artist? Can classical music be called Black music, or White music? Should we demarcate music in this way, or is it that the politics is different if we are talking about being excluded from a space rather than being appropriated in 'our' space? Surely, if I followed this logic of White and Black music, I would end up talking myself out of a job?

For me, these arguments about the identity of music couldn't be as simple and clear-cut as they seemed on the surface, and I had always had to dig deeper and think harder. We are always in a nexus of competing traditions as artists and there is a dysfunctional relationship between self-expression and trespass. I had fought, and keep fighting, to prove myself as a classical musician, and was I really an unwelcome and inappropriate stranger here?

One approach is to look at the history of classical music and closely examine claims made – in its favour or against it – as a bastion of White, Western tradition, owned by a lineage of illustrious musicians who defined its terms, making it their territory. In this story, I could only ever be indulging in role play and imitation as a classical performer. I could only ever be taking the job away from the White musician who should be there in my place. Who did I think I was?

As soon as we look seriously at the history of classical music, we see the gaps where Black composers and musicians used to be, visible and successful, creating and transforming the art they were part of and in which they were championed. I'm continually astonished at just how radical their disappearance was from the canon and how devastatingly complete a deliberate policy of forgetting can be. We are the history we tell ourselves and British, European, American and Western identity depends on stories that cement its dominant ideologies. If classical music is to be claimed as the jealously guarded mainland of White music, the Black musicians that were part and parcel of its multifaceted, multiracial, Western story, have to be expunged.

These musicians were never presented as anything more than scribbles in the margins, lesser and less skilled artists who were never truly movers and shakers in a world alien to their sensibilities and training. But it's becoming clearer just how influential many of them were and how well they were known and admired. So how can they have been purged so effectively from the official histories of classical music, and what does that say about the vulnerability of Black artistic legacies?

The more we look the more we uncover important Black composers and performers who were very influential and indeed famous and celebrated in their day – even relatively recently – and have been silenced, as though they never existed. Like the pages of Western history, what is Western is a constantly retold narrative, wiped bleach-clean of the diverse tales that have always threaded through and even created it.

I was entranced to discover the works of Samuel Coleridge-Taylor, the composer whose fame was at its height in the world of the early twentieth century, particularly in the UK and the USA. He was born in 1875 and died at the young age of thirty-seven in Croydon, South London in 1912. His father, like one of my grandfathers, was from Sierra Leone, West Africa, and his mother was English. Having graduated as a prodigy from the Royal College of Music he used, in many of his works, the traditional melodies and idioms associated with his own Black identity as the life force for his classical compositions. Using African-American spirituals he wrote a series of piano arrangements which brought the songs of the slaves into classical music and created something new.[1]

This has always been part of the tradition of classical composition. Coleridge-Taylor himself points out in his introduction to Twenty-Four Negro Melodies Op. 59: 'What Brahms has done for the Hungarian folk-music, Dvořák for the Bohemian, and Grieg for the Norwegian, I have tried to do for Negro melodies.' Dvořák included 'negro melodies' in his New World Symphony, influenced by a Black student, Henry Burleigh, at the New York conservatory where he worked. By doing this, Dvořák raised the visibility and perceived value of African-American music and infused a stirring historical and contemporary vitality into the classical symphony. This borrowing between folk and classical has long been common practice among classical composers, from Mozart to Liszt to Shostakovich. There is nothing marginal about Coleridge-Taylor's music, unless spirituals are less 'folk' than Hungarian Gypsy music.

Coleridge-Taylor's stunning success as a composer is astonishing given the obscurity that cloaked his reputation from the Second World War onwards. Perhaps the most well-known English composer from this period is Edward Elgar, and his towering reputation and music have become synonymous with a form of English or British patriotism. What has endured is a polished view of Elgar and his music over and above Coleridge-Taylor who was, in many ways, Elgar's more beloved and successful contemporary. The fact that Coleridge-Taylor was taken out of print and largely dropped from classical programming is not as straightforward as it seems on the surface. The reinstatement of Coleridge-Taylor's legacy by putting his work back into regular concert hall repertoire, and reintroducing him to audiences, allows us to see how paths of connection and conversation that were always there can be deliberately shrouded by time and choice. Coleridge-Taylor borrowed from Henry Longfellow, the abolitionist English poet, as well as Paul Laurence Dunbar, the African-American poet. He was mentored by Elgar and had close friendships with Vaughan Williams and Holst. He was welcomed with open arms and feted in the USA, given an audience with President Roosevelt in the White House, and was the first Black man there to conduct a White orchestra. In London, he was hugely famous, even after his death, his music having been performed at the Proms an amazing 116 times between 1898 and 1939.

But why am I amazed? Maybe it's because of epitaphs and labels that stick. Joseph Bologne, the exciting composer, violinist, fencer and soldier of eighteenth-century France, born in the colony of Guadeloupe and fantastically famous in Europe, adored by Marie Antoinette and looked up to by Mozart, regularly has his reputation reduced to the 'Black Mozart'.[2] Likewise, Coleridge-Taylor bears the title 'Black Mahler'. It doesn't matter how well-known, beautiful or successful the work is. If a composer, musician, social or political figure, statesman or intellect, is Black, that Blackness is a burden. And sometimes that burden can obscure everything else about them.

There are many other Black classical composers and performers who we are either rediscovering or have yet to discover in many Western countries. Apart from Joseph Bologne, the Chevalier de Saint-Georges, whose oeuvre of music – violin concertos, string quartets, sinfonia concertante, violin duets, sonatas, symphonies and comic opera – is substantial and exquisite, there are also women musicians whose under-appreciation and lack of visibility as classical artists is extraordinary. Florence Price, whose piano concerto has been recorded by my sister Jeneba with Chineke! Orchestra, was a prolific composer and pianist whose work has been largely unpreserved.[3] The musicologist Samantha Ege has written about and recorded the work of Florence Price, becoming a recognized expert on this Black woman composer who was the first to have a symphony, her Symphony in E Minor, performed by a major American orchestra when it was played in 1933 by the Chicago Symphony.[4] When I listen to Jeneba's recording, I hear the jazz and ragtime of African-American music, and the powerful resonance of spirituals. But next to the humming of slaves and the African dance rhythms of Juba, I also hear the influence of late Romanticism. Here is Liszt next to Scott Joplin, a modern USA next to the European and African traditions that create Western music.

It matters to my brother, sisters and me that this music is played. Isata has recorded Coleridge-Taylor next to George Gershwin, Earl Wild, Samuel Barber, Amy Beach, Aaron Copland and African-American spirituals.[5] I write this list because the contextuality of Black music is often forgotten. It exists as part of the formation, constitution, ever-changing enrichment of classical music. It *is* classical music and classical exists on the fluid borders of jazz, spirituals, folk and other forms of history and influence as dynamically as any music.

It matters to us that the music and stories of people we identify with is played by us. Braimah appeared in Bill Barclay's play *The Chevalier* at Snape Maltings and in London's St Martin-in-the-Fields in 2023 (with the London Philharmonic Orchestra) playing the music of Joseph Bologne within the costumed story of his life. We have performed the spiritual *Deep River*, arranged by us from Coleridge-Taylor's piano transcripts for our family trio and septet, many times. It matters because the act of placing ourselves at the centre of the music we love, in the shoes and with the music of those who share our identity in these particular, contested ways, is powerful. The implicit or explicit label of 'marginal' or alien for Black classical artists is a constant pressure and those moments where we can fit within the music that – by its origins – is incontestably ours is a refutation.

Nina Simone, famously associated with the 'Black music' of gospel, blues, jazz and R & B, was at heart, and by training and ambition, a classical pianist. She enrolled at the Juilliard School of Music in New York and a year later auditioned for a scholarship place at the Curtis Institute of Music. It seems clear that this period of punishing hard work, pledging her time, energy and love to her craft and giving a well-received audition, was one of the most important periods of her life. The rejection she received from Curtis changed her life and broke her heart. Her classical training gave her the phenomenal technique as well as the discipline and phrasing she kept with her in subsequent years, but she was banished from the territory and legacy of classical music from then on. Her words in the documentary *What Happened, Miss*

Simone? still haunt me: 'I knew I was good enough, but they turned me down. And it took me about six months to realize it was because I was Black. I never really got over that jolt of racism at the time.'[6]

That 'jolt of racism' is the unspeakable moment we mostly keep to ourselves. The silencing of our voices is part of our ticket into this hallowed region of classical music, even though our music has always been part of its existence.

But does that mean that only Black musicians should now be playing Black classical music? I am always asked, when on concert tour, why I don't have more music by Black composers in my repertoire. Isata is always asked why she doesn't have whole programmes of women composers, or Black women composers. If we want to make Black and women composers central to the classical repertoire, it can't only be Black and women musicians who play their work. I play music that I love, that I engage with, that speaks to me, that I want to play. If we, as Black and/or women musicians, are pushed into a restrictive identity politics with the kind of music we are permitted to play, then White and male musicians get to play . . . everything else? And that 'everything else' is then, still, seen as outside any identity restrictions, just 'good', just 'classical', just 'the real thing'. And nothing changes.

I want to play music by women composers, by Russian, Jewish, German, French, Brazilian, Spanish composers, without having to 'be' any of them. Music transcends nationality, race and gender, but that doesn't mean these issues are not profoundly important, and serious. They are important because of the way these identities are used to exclude and marginalize those who are already disadvantaged. However, the responsibility to decolonize the classical music canon rests on all our shoulders and not just on those who have already been left out for far too long.

My passion for composing and arranging, allowing my identity, my background, my own cultural influences to be expressed, is an important way for me to bring my whole self into the music I play. I will often arrange the music of Bob Marley, or Aretha Franklin, or many others from outside the classical repertoire, and play their music as an encore, or as a recording. I often compose using idioms from different traditions that speak to me or have influenced me in a way I find inspiring or moving. It seems to me that the energy I bring from my own background is vital to the classical music world, the same way I see orchestras like Chineke! as bringing something dynamic into classical music.

Musicians bring new ideas, new influences, new ways of playing, of protesting, of emoting, of remembering into music – and how much more explosive and progressive that can be if musicians themselves come from different backgrounds and experiences.

But music from outside the canon, or rather, in the

case of a lot of rediscovered Black composition, music that was originally in the canon and was then denied its place, deserves the same scholarship, time, love and serious contemplation as Elgar's cello concerto or Mozart's Requiem. Playing 'Black' classical music as though it speaks for itself in its own thin, decontextualized form, diminishes it next to the works seen as 'central' to the genre.

What is the future of classical music? That depends on what happens with music education, and also what happens with politics in wider society. There is a fraught battle being waged over culture, race, class and identity, and it's being waged in our schools, in the media and in our creative and performing arts industries. My mission is to refute the stereotypes we are being forced to confront, to resist accepting that the status quo is somehow inevitable, and constantly to question the ownership and the identity of the music I am determined to keep playing.

If I refer back to my discussions with other Black musicians in 2020, I realize that all these arguments are nuanced and specific. We can talk about the exploitation of Black music in particular circumstances, and we can refuse what these labels mean in others. The end of this sentence: 'This is Black music so therefore . . .' is not and should not be always the same, just as the beginning of the sentence: 'This is Black music . . .' has to be contested at different times and in different places. My place as a British musician needs always to be claimed and reclaimed along with an unrelenting and unrepentant interrogation of what 'British' means. Our place is already in the story, and we all belong in its history. But, crucially, our perspectives, feelings, sufferings and losses are different from each other. I want to listen to the many voices within classical music that were always there and that still define the landscape. If we don't allow these voices in the room or we silence them when they are there, we risk the desiccation of the genre we love.

I have an example that goes to the tender core of these issues. It's an example so timely and immediate it's become explosive, and several of us have been burnt on approach. I appeared on the BBC Radio 4 programme *Desert Island Discs* in January 2024. When the host, Lauren Laverne, asked me whether I thought 'Rule, Britannia!' should be dropped from the Last Night of the Proms repertoire, I said yes. There are a few things that are guaranteed to spark the volcano of racism that bubbles underground in the UK, and this is one of them. Many people outside the UK were frankly bemused by the rage I had quietly stoked, and could afford an amused and rather wry glance at it all, but from inside the atmosphere was toxic.

I am a passionate supporter of the BBC Proms. Its

series of concerts are a testament to the strength and
creativity of live classical music, and I treasure the
significance of this summer festival and its continuing
legacy. A number of the concerts are televised but it's
always been the case that the Last Night is reserved for
the showcase, prime-time slot. It's a night where Britishness is proudly exhibited in all its joy, pomp and
ceremony. We hear music from around the UK – from
Wales, Scotland and Ireland – sea shanties from Britain's
island traditions, and compositions new and old. A lot
of the repertoire is interchangeable and can be altered,
dependent upon the choice of musicians and programme planners, reflecting the passions or obsessions
of the day. One section, however, has become somehow
immovable, and an ice-hard determination to preserve
its place has settled around it. It's a moment that most
musicians and those who decide the repertoire would
dearly love to leave behind as a rather embarrassing
reminder of a Britishness that celebrates imperial glory
and subjugation. It's a moment which acts to turn away
many who themselves, and their relatives and ascend-
ants, are on the wrong side of that history.

The angry and somewhat baffling energy directed at
retaining 'Rule, Britannia!' seems to rest on the idea that
here *is* Britishness, here *is* Englishness. Here are the root
and proof of 'our' nationalist pride, and this is who 'we'
are. It makes no odds – and seems utterly enraging to

the defenders of this song – that there are many of us who don't fit into that 'we', or who feel profoundly and aggressively attacked by it.

I had been honoured to perform at the Last Night the summer before. I loved playing and collaborating with the incredible Norwegian soprano Lise Davidsen, and the Last Night is a wonderful culmination of the world-class, exciting, innovative, inclusive and exceptional concerts in the weeks that precede it. For Lise, as a Norwegian, there was nothing controversial about the lyrics of 'Rule, Britannia!' or the charged sentiment within it, but for me, the situation was very different. I was not required to be onstage for its rowdy, raucous and heated rendition, the entire – almost entire – Royal Albert Hall of five thousand people roaring the lines: 'Rule, Britannia! Britannia, rule the waves! Britons never, never, never will be slaves.' Using the words from a 1740 poem, 'Rule Britannia' by James Thomson, and set to music by Thomas Arne in the same year, it is a composition tied to a particular kind of patriotism. Its vigour and intent were born in Britain's burgeoning slave trade and at the height of its thundering imperialism.

I wasn't asked on the radio to give my historical analysis of the song, but to explain how I felt and could have felt being in the room while the song was belted out, unapologetically and rousingly, all around me. I had chosen to remain backstage for this moment because, I explained, it made me – and many others – feel uncomfortable. I said no more, but hoped my response was valid because honest. It was entirely true, and mattered, not just to me, but to whole groups of British people who felt we had a stake in a definition of Britishness. If our inclusion meant we should happily boast that we were not people who could be enslaved or subjugated by navy or army, we were radically *not* included. For my family, as descendants of slaves, or born in colonies, none of this was distant history.

All my siblings and both my parents, loyal and wanting to support me, had been unable to escape their seats in the auditorium and sat, weak-kneed and heads bowed, as crowds stood and shout-sang their victorious nationhood around them. Most of my family were in tears by the end, and all of them were miserable and frightened.

My truthful and understated remark on *Desert Island Discs*, that the song made many of us 'uncomfortable' was greeted with an uproarious wave of censure and horror against me in the media, and an unguarded uprising of racist bile on social media. People called for me to be 'tagged, flogged and deported', to 'go back home' and to 'keep my n***er mouth shut'. Extreme, inflammatory reactions like these operate on the same spectrum as the indignant, offended responses I also received. It didn't matter how I felt, or how non-White people feel. It didn't matter that we suffered, were excluded or frightened by a nationalism we couldn't share. If we wanted to stay at the centre and apex of our most prestigious classical music festival, proudly broadcast nationally on Saturday evening television and radio, our voices had to be fervently and bitterly silenced.

Then if playing classical music is an exercise in self-denial, role play and dishonesty, so many of us remain, like Nina Simone, on the outside.

Coda: On Hope and Change

I am infused with hope and belief that the future of classical music is bright. There are so many reasons to be optimistic. Look, for example, at Errollyn Wallen, the current Master of the King's Music, appointed in 2024. She was also the first Black woman composer to win the Ivor Novello Award and to have her work featured at the BBC Proms. More music by Black and women composers, and by new composers, is being heard at the Proms and in concerts with major orchestras. The 2024 BBC Proms had record-breaking sales for its concert tickets, with audience numbers projected from its first weekend of sales up by almost 36 per cent from the year before, pointing to a growing engagement in classical music at the UK's biggest classical music festival.[1] This enduring and even growing emphasis on live audience numbers, with many Proms concerts in 2024 selling out, exists alongside the fact that the BBC broadcasts every concert on BBC Radio 3, and many of the concerts on BBC television absolutely free.

My brother and sisters, who like me should statistically have been unlikely to become classical musicians, also have highly successful careers, performing and recording internationally on piano, violin and cello. More music by Black and women composers, and by new composers, is available for all of us to play and is being commissioned and heard at the Proms and in concerts with major orchestras. The banner of classical music is being carried by a wave of exciting young classical musicians from, for example, the Sphinx Organization, based in Detroit, USA, or the Simón Bolívar Symphony Orchestra in Venezuela. Projects for young players, like the Antigua and Barbuda Youth Symphony Orchestra, or the National Children's Orchestra of Great Britain, and initiatives like Black Lives in Music, to name just a few, are all inspiring an ever-changing and energetic engagement with classical music for everyone.

Music has always been reflective of the changes, pre-occupations and contentions of the times, but also its possibilities. Who classical musicians and composers are, who is in the audience and what constitutes the repertoire, all these are determined by social and political choices. They are determined by what we value – and whether that includes our children, our elderly, our disadvantaged, our marginalized. The future of music itself will emerge from our ability to be creative and to express ourselves. It depends on how we are heard. I believe that the present, and the future, rely on how we construct the past. History, including the history of music, is a contested territory in which we all have a stake, and borders are ever debated, shifted and dissolved.

Classical music is my identity and my self-definition. I

have worked hard to learn to be articulate in its language, and there is endlessly more to explore, whether already written or yet to exist. I will continue to collaborate, to listen and to create, interpreting, arranging and making anew. Our job as musicians is to reach those who are still out of range, and to move, surprise and persuade those already here. What I do is out of love. It is the will to communicate and to make connections that drives us all. And music is my art and my home.

Reprise

Recordings I'd recommend to anyone, whether classical
music connoisseur or first-time listener:

Sergei Rachmaninov: Piano Concerto No. 2
Sergei Rachmaninov (piano), Leopold Stokowski (conductor), Philadelphia Orchestra (RCA)

Frank Bridge: Sonata for Cello and Piano
Steven Isserlis (cello), Connie Shih (piano), *The Cello in
Wartime* (BIS Records)

Tom Poster and Elena Urioste: *From Brighton to Brooklyn*
(Chandos)

Edmund Finnis: String Quartets 1 and 2
Manchester Collective, *Shades* (Bedroom Community)

Haydn: String Quartets, Op. 20 ('Sun' Quartets)
(Hyperion Records)

Brahms: Cello and Piano Sonatas
Daniel Barenboim and Jacqueline du Pré (Warner Classics)

Mozart: Symphony No. 40
Sándor Végh (conductor), Camerata Salzburg (Sony)

Acknowledgements

In writing this book, I have been constantly aware that I did not get here alone, and that everything I have achieved has been as part of a family, a community and a network of friends, teachers and mentors. Any potential I may have shown in music has been nurtured, encouraged and taught by the people around me.

Musicians are listened to before they can be heard, tutored before they can perform, and inspired before they themselves can inspire others. I am a product of the love, faith and expectation of those who have brought me up, shared my childhood, offered me friendship and showed me the discipline and the artistry of music. I have been lucky, but my luck has been in the effort, determination and generosity of others, and I am endlessly thankful.

Throughout the pages of this book, I have named teachers and friends who have helped me in my life and in my music. Here, I would like to add my wonderful manager, Kathryn Enticott, who has never stopped believing in me and who has been by my side from the very beginning of my career as a cellist. From the time when I was still a teenage boy, Kathryn's friendship and guidance have been invaluable.

ACKNOWLEDGEMENTS

Thank you to my literary agent, Todd Schuster, and to my editor, Ella Harold, whose enthusiasm and support for this book have kept me going.

My mother, Kadiatu Kanneh-Mason, has been a significant sounding-board for many of my insights and arguments, engaging me in conversation and discussion, and helping me to think through the issues that preoccupy me. This book has come into being as a collaboration between us, and we have worked very closely together. My thanks go to her for her deep interest and involvement with the writing of this project.

My hope is that the passion I have for music has run deep into every sentence and every page of this book. My conviction is that music is an art, a skill and a gift, and also that it is the right of every child and of every adult. Music is human, transformative, everyday and extraordinary. Music is powerful.

Notes

3. Education and Opportunity

1 See Heidi Ashton, 'Cutting the STEM of future skills: Beyond the STEM vs art dichotomy in England', *Arts and Humanities in Higher Education*, 2023, Vol. 22(2) 148–163.

2 See Black Lives in Music report, September 2021: 'Being Black in the UK Music Industry'.

3 The statistics are readily available and eloquent. For example, the report 'Equality and Diversity in the Classical Music Profession' by Dr Christina Scharff from King's College London (February 2015) cited data from 2014 across seventeen orchestras which found that 1.7 per cent of orchestral players 'could be identified from a black and minority ethnic background'. In 2021 the Arts Council England published 'Creating a More Inclusive Classical Music: A study of the English orchestral workforce and the current routes to joining it'. This states: 'Black or Black British musicians are underrepresented at each stage within elite training opportunities. As the training stages progress, the overall intake becomes less ethnically diverse.' Looking at the classical music profession, the outcome is evident: 'Amongst the orchestral workforce in England only

between 3–6% were Black, Asian or from other ethnically diverse groups.' This doesn't necessarily represent a rise from the 2014 King's College data, of course, but a wider remit.

4 Bridget Whyte and Deborah Annetts, 'Reflections on Music Hubs', Cultural Learning Alliance, 22 July 2024.

5 Ofsted is the Office for Standards in Education, Children's Services and Skills and carries out school inspections. Ofsted has jurisdiction only in England. Estyn is the equivalent for Wales; for Scotland, it's Education Scotland, and for Northern Ireland it's the Education and Training Inspectorate.

6 Julian Lloyd Webber, *The Strad*, 28 June 2018.

7 Jess Gillam, *Guardian*, 10 February 2019.

8 Sharma, Samata R. and Silbersweig, David, 'Setting the Stage: Neurobiological Effects of Music on the Brain', 2018.

9 Crossroads of Music and Medicine 6. White Paper published 1 June 2018.

10 Also, the psychology journal *Frontiers* has published a research topic on 'The Impact of Music on Human Development and Well-Being' with global reach, examining the psychological, neurological, therapeutic and physical effects of music learning and activity. *Frontiers*, 17 June 2020, Vol. II, https://doi.org/10.3389/fpsyg.2020.01246.

11 In addition, amongst a wealth of research I could draw on, the University of Southern California *Science Daily* (18 January 2023) published these findings: 'The latest USC

research on the impact of music education shows that for adolescents, the benefits appear to extend beyond a surge in neural connections in their brains. It actually boosts their wellbeing.'

12 Gov.UK. Published under the 2019 to 2022 Johnson Conservative government, 25 June 2022. Last updated 15 May 2024.

13 The Independent Society of Musicians, Musicians' Union and Music Mark in a letter to Gillian Keegan, Secretary of State for Education, December 2023.

14 I realize I've introduced more concepts from the English education system that stand like towering monoliths over music. Like core and STEM subjects, the English Baccalaureate, or EBacc (beloved of current education policy – which is always, hopefully, subject to change) despises music as a subject and refuses to include it. The Department of Education guidance (updated 20 August 2019) summarizes this ideal secondary school curriculum as: 'a set of subjects at GCSE that keeps young people's options open for further study and future careers'. The EBacc is: 'English language and literature, maths, the sciences, geography or history, a language' (ancient or modern). But music is entirely unnecessary. Progress 8 and Attainment 8 describe the measures used to make schools accountable for pupils' attainment across subjects, but these subjects are, of course, circumscribed by the EBacc, ghosting music and making maths 'double-weighted'.

15 Richard Morrison, *The Times*, 30 June 2022.
16 Dr Ally Daubney, in her keynote address for Westminster Education Forum, 26 October 2023: 'The Current State of Music Education and the Impact of the National Plan for Music Education'.

4. Equality or Quality?

1 BBC Radio 4, *Desert Island Discs*, 21 January 2024.

5. Relevance and Power

1 '10 Classical Music Pieces in Video Games', Joshua Zinn, 19 June 2015, Houston Public Media. Or, for the inspiration of video game music in classical music, see 'Video Games Inspire a Generation of Classical Music Fans', in Mat Ombler, *Wired*, 4 November 2021.
2 BBC Radio 3, *Music Matters: Land Without Music*, 6 April 2024.
3 BBC Radio 4, *Front Row*, 10 April 2024.
4 'Chechnya Forbids Music Outside 80–116 BPM Tempo', *Moscow Times*, 5 April 2024. See also 'Chechnya Bans Dance Music that is Either Too Fast or Too Slow', Philip Oltermann, *Guardian*, 9 April 2024.
5 *Moscow Times*, 5 April 2024.

6 Richard Morrison, *The Times*, 15 August 2024: 'We Cut Arts Funding but Spent £4m on Each Olympic Medal. Is That Fair?'

7 'First 30 years – personal memories'. This personal history was produced by founder member Jo Bucklow (with help from others) for the thirtieth anniversary concert in 2018.

6. Music and Identity

1 'Passions: Chi-chi Nwanoku on Samuel Coleridge-Taylor', Maclarty Brown Media, Sky Arts, 28 November 2017. See also *Samuel Coleridge-Taylor: A Musical Life*, Jeffrey Green, Routledge, 2011.

2 See Bill Barclay's play *The Chevalier*, which was performed at Snape Maltings on 19 March 2023, and St Martin-in-the-Fields on 21 March 2023, with the London Philharmonic Orchestra and my brother, Braimah, as violinist Joseph Bologne.

3 *Florence Price*, Chineke! Orchestra, featuring Jeneba Kanneh-Mason, Decca Classics, 2023.

4 See Samantha Ege: *South Side Impresarios: How Race Women Transformed Chicago's Classical Music Scene*, University of Illinois Press, 2024. Also, Samantha Ege and A. Kori Hill, eds, *The Cambridge Companion to Florence B. Price*, Cambridge University Press, 2024. And also, '"Their Music

Lit a Fire in Me": Hearing the voices of three neglected composers gave me my own', Samantha Ege, *Guardian*, 19 November 2021.

5 Decca Classics, 2021.

6 *What Happened, Miss Simone?* Documentary directed by Liz Garbus, Netflix, 26 June 2015.

Coda: On Hope and Change

1 BBC Media Centre, 20 May 2024.